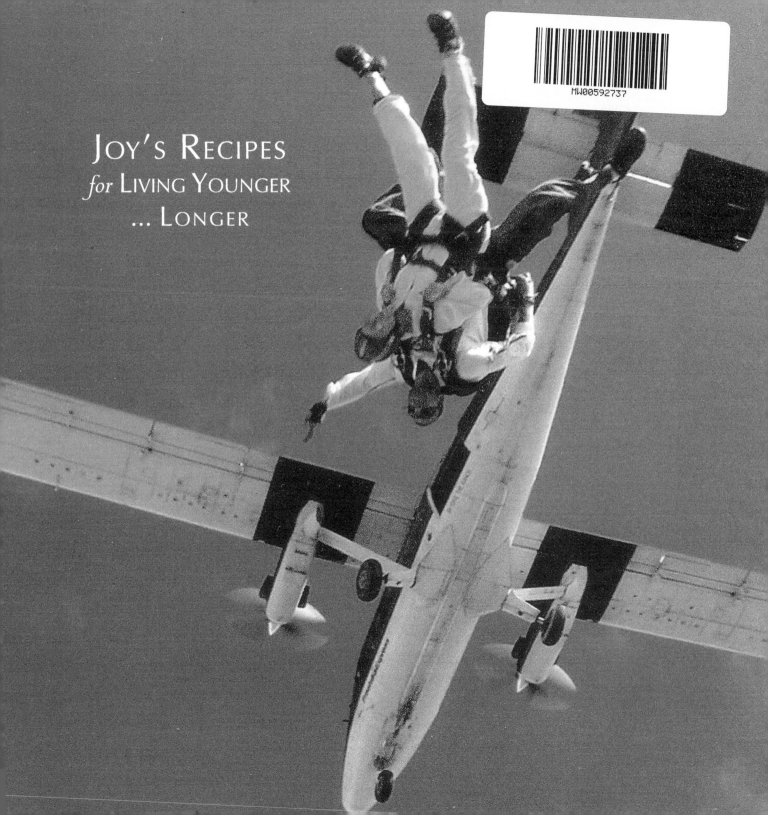

JOY'S RECIPES
for LIVING YOUNGER
... LONGER

MW00592737

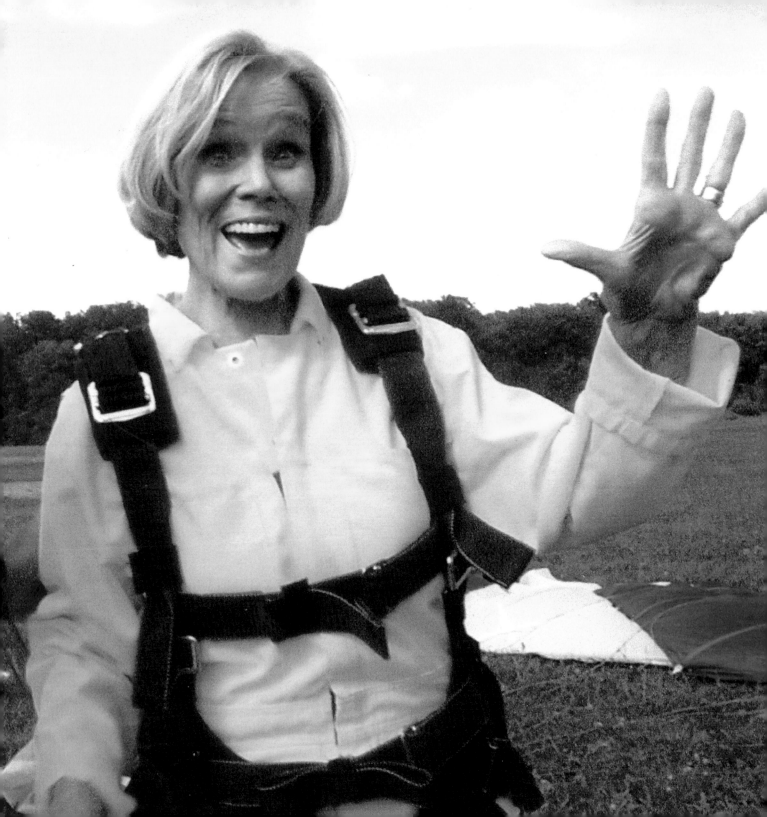

Joy's Recipes
for Living Younger ... *Longer*

An Eighty-Something Beauty Reveals Her Secrets

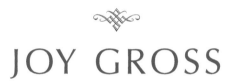

Joy Gross

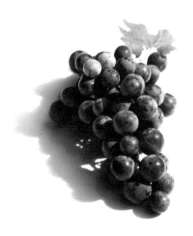

Epigraph Books
Rhinebeck, New York

Printed in the United States of America

Photographs by Ron Reeves
www.ronreeves.com

Book and cover design by Georgia Dent

Dishware, cookware, cutlery and linens courtesy of:
bluecashew
Kitchen Pharmacy
6423 Montgomery Street, Suite 3
Rhinebeck NY 12572
845.876.1117
www.bluecashew.com

Library of Congress Control Number: 2010940185
ISBN: 978-0-9830517-2-5

Epigraph Books
27 Lamoree Road
Rhinebeck, New York 12572
www.epigraphPS.com
USA 845.876.4861

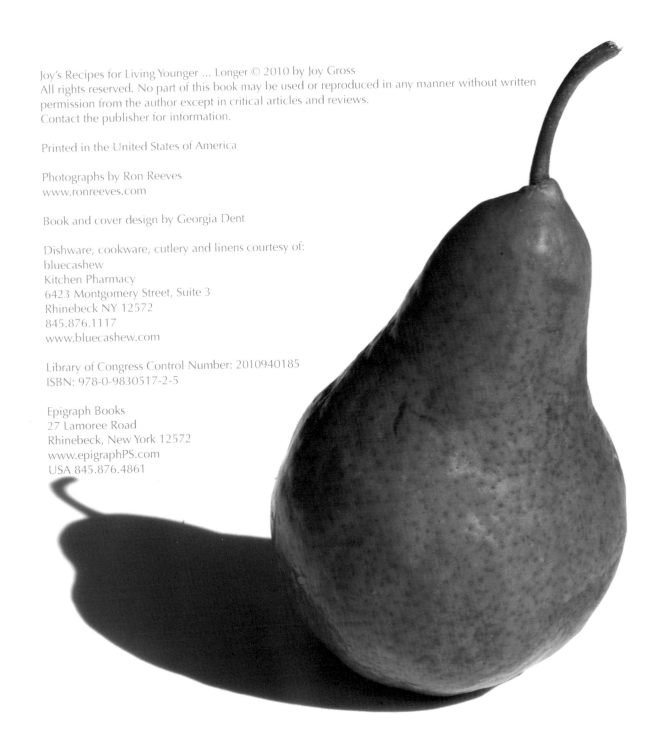

To my five children,
Louis, David, Betsy, Debbie, and Wendy

And to my five grandchildren,
Cara, Emma, Matthew, Eric, and Sarah

And to my great-granddaughter, Seychelle

And to my surrogate granddaughter, Bigi

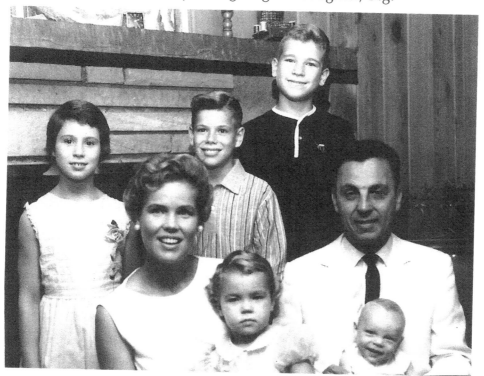

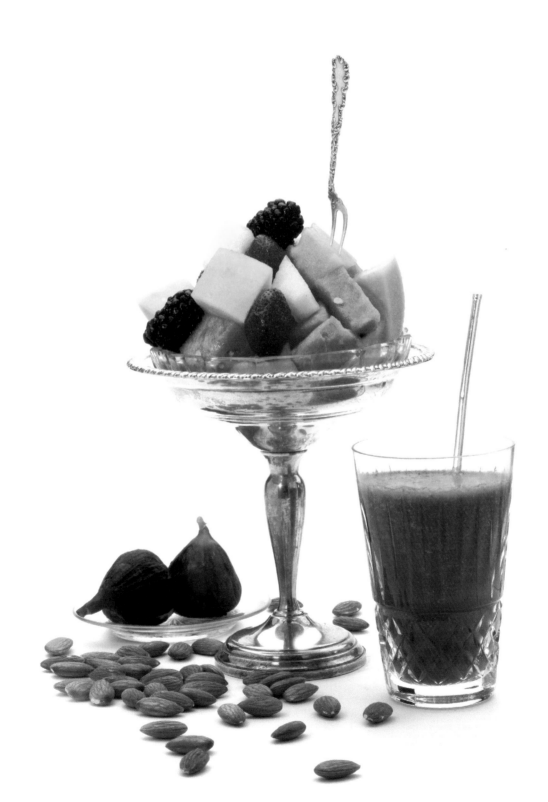

What you put into your body has an immediate effect. It makes a difference in how you look, how you feel, and how quickly you age. By changing to a new way of eating and thinking—by making it easier for your ever-faithful and hardworking cells to do their job—you can change your body and your world.

—Joy Gross

The greatest courage comes from the highest conviction.

—Helen Keller

We hold on to our bad habits because we are not really committed to grow and we need an excuse for our failures.

—David Viscott, M.D.

The health, strength, youth, growth, and preservation of the body depend upon a certain fixed degree of alkalinity. Old age is a disease which has not yet taken on organic form. It is the result of … acid waste accumulation.

—Herbert M. Shelton, N.D., D.C.

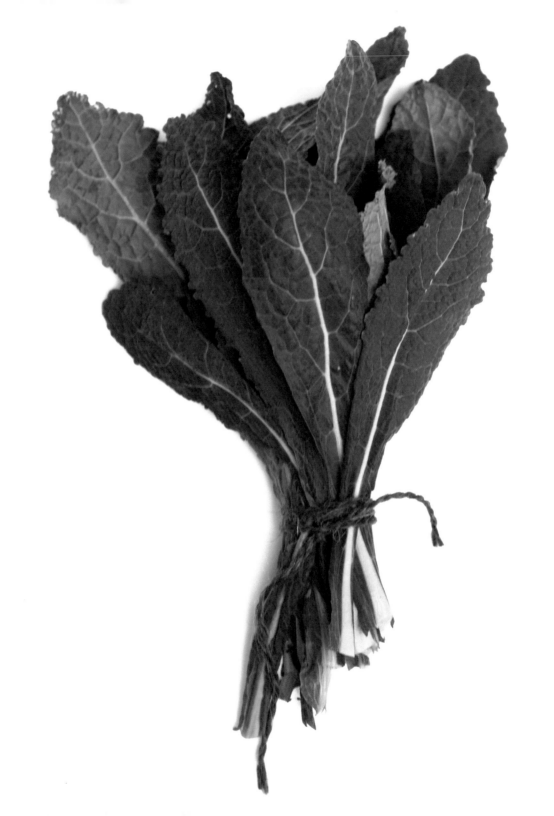

CONTENTS

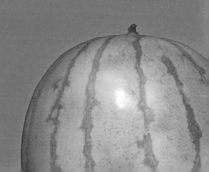

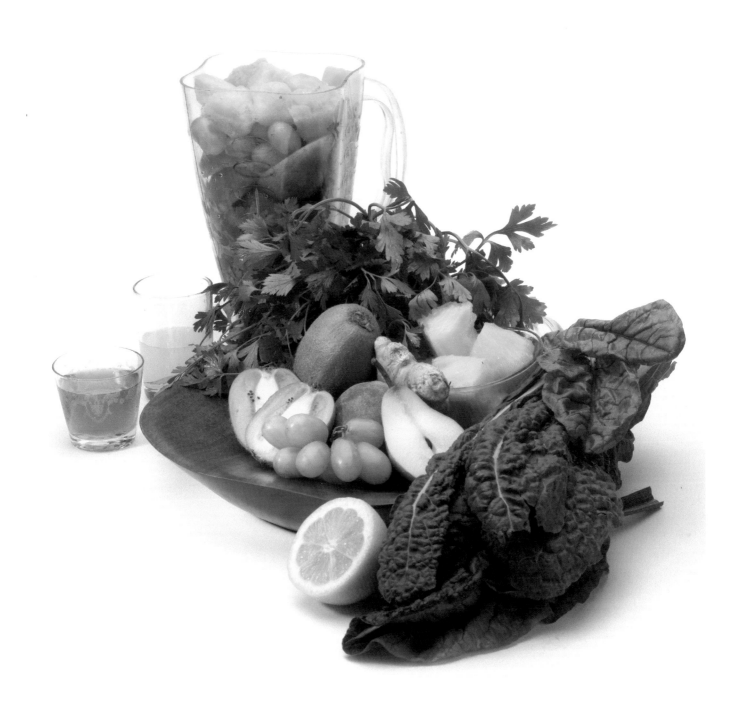

THE WAY TO LIVE
YOUNGER... LONGER

Have you arrived at that day of reckoning when you look in the mirror and find yourself admitting, "I don't like the way I look. I don't like the way I feel. I wish I could start over again!"

Well, you can.

My experiences, and those of many others, have proven that when you change your diet and institute healthful practices in your life, you will end up looking and feeling brand new. You can revolutionize your entire approach to living.

What I will be sharing with you in this book is based on my firsthand experience, which includes working with tens of thousands of guests who came to my Pawling Health Manor in upstate New York for over three decades.

The Manor's clients included such luminous actresses as Veronica Lake, Jessica Tandy, Shelley Winters, and Cicely Tyson; jazz giants Miles Davis and Charlie Mingus; comedian Jerry Stiller; opera star Grace Bumbry; Yankees owner George Steinbrenner; bestselling novelist Judith Rossner; and world-renowned choreographer Alvin Ailey.

The health secrets for which these celebrities paid tens of thousands of dollars are revealed to you in this book. More than ever, I want to share with you a bit of my health philosophy, along with some great plant-based recipes—including pictures—to make it easier and more exciting for you. It's inspiring to

me, as I eat and live for the vibrant health I enjoy, to know that my way is also the better way for our animal friends and for the planet.

You will learn that health is wholeness. The most important thing I discovered—over sixty-five years ago—is that life is based on awesome immutable laws, and ignorance of those laws does not excuse anyone from suffering the consequences of breaking them.

But if you're willing to accept the Laws of Life, and integrate them into your daily behavior, they will keep you well, young, and beautiful.

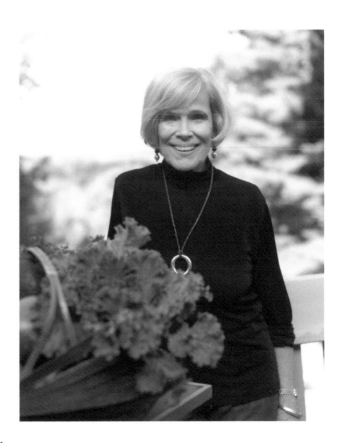

MY STORY

When folks learn that I've been a vegetarian, mostly vegan, for almost seventy years, they are curious to know why. I was so far ahead of the times!

I am positive that had I not had serious health problems I would have never chosen that path. I grew up in the little town of Hazelwood, North Carolina, nestled high in the Blue Ridge mountains. My father, a Presbyterian minister, was pastor of a quaint little white-steepled church next door to the manse where we lived. Daddy had grown up in western Kentucky and Mother in Los Angeles; they'd met at a Bible Institute in LA. I was their first child.

When I was five years old, my mother became friends with a young widow, Helen, who had moved next door. They would chat while watching us children play; and one day Helen told Mother about a new diet she'd started—the Hay Diet, originated by William Howard Hay, M.D.

Mother became interested and decided to give it a try, not only for herself but for the entire family, which by now included my brother Owen. Out went the fried chicken (except when we had company) and white bread, ice cream, and just about all my favorite foods.

Except for Mother, we hated the diet. All white sugar and white flour products were banned. Meat was allowed only sparingly.

Just as depressing was a new concept: food combining. We weren't supposed to eat starches with acids—for example, orange juice with toast. We also had to cut out starches with protein—for instance, bread and cheese, or cereal with milk. Even today, food combining has its adherents and its skeptics. I myself am careful about mixing foods together because different foods require different enzymatic action in the digestive process.

A recommended way to start the day was by drinking a tall glass of hot water with fresh lemon juice. And since Mother was the "boss," we were her prisoners.

Some time later Helen told Mother about a health retreat that she had stayed at in Hendersonville. It was called the Health School, run by a Dr. Oliver Dahl. Helen had undergone a water fast to detoxify her system. Mother got excited about the idea and decided she too needed to go there, both to lose some weight and to get healthier.

Off she went, leaving Daddy, Owen, and me to fend for ourselves for an entire month. While she was gone, Daddy did the shopping and made the meals. He restored some of the bygone goodies to the pantry. He made fried chicken and hot dogs for us. We drank ginger ale and Coca-Cola with our meals, and we ate bacon and eggs for breakfast.

When Mother came back to us, she was thinner and running over with renewed enthusiasm for the new diet. The first night home

2

she made eggplant steaks and a huge green salad. Daddy helped himself to a big slice of eggplant, wadded it into a ball in the palm of his hand, and—having been a baseball player in his younger years—wound up and made the pitch … toward the coal bucket across the room. It made a perfect landing!

When I was seven, my sister Gennie was born. She hated the new diet, too, as early as the tender age of three—and was a more brazen rebel than either Owen or I dared to be. She would run through the neighborhood looking for handouts. She'd knock on a neighbor's door. "I'm hungry," she'd say. Gennie would always be invited in and offered goodies such as cookies and cake, white bread sandwiches, and ice cream.

I managed to sneak in quite a bit of contraband by trading school lunches (mine was usually an apple or a banana and a thermos of raw milk) for peanut butter and jelly on white bread. I saved my nickels and pennies for Hershey's kisses and Cokes at the corner store.

Owen and I also became devious about getting the goodies to which we felt entitled. For instance, one sunny afternoon we went next door to Mrs. McElroy's with a measuring cup. I knocked and, when Mrs. McElroy opened the door, held forth the cup as Owen and I said in unison, "Our mother wants to borrow a cup of white sugar!" She looked at us with suspicion but took the cup and handed it back filled to the brim with sparkling white sugar. We carefully made our way back behind our house, around the front of the church next door, climbed the stone stairway to the secluded porch, huddled down into a corner and, sharing the one teaspoon we'd thoughtfully brought along, took turns devouring the contents of the cup. We had triumphed over Helen, Mother, Dr. Hay, and Dr. Dahl.

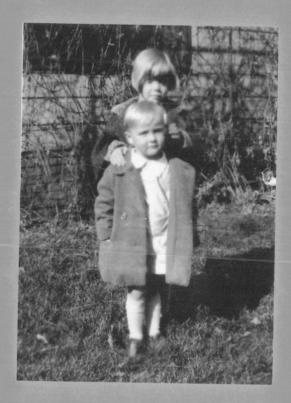

The Skin Problem

For as long as I can remember, I had a mild problem with psoriasis. When I was nine, it got worse. And the more contraband I managed to sneak into my diet, the worse it got. The bumps in my scalp got bumpier and, when I scratched them, bloodier.

Besides the psoriasis, I was prone to anything that could go wrong with skin. I frequently developed styes in the corner of my eyes. Carbuncles and boils would occasionally manifest themselves. It was embarrassing and painful.

Mother made an appointment with a dermatologist. Dr. Whitehead made the diagnosis. "Joy has psoriasis. There's no known cause and no known cure. She'll just have to learn to live with it." And that was that. His only advice was to soften the scabs with baby oil—which made me look like a wet-head. I was doomed, or so it seemed.

Although my psoriasis was somewhat better when I followed Mother's dietary rules, I still felt compelled to sneak in a significant amount of contraband. When I was thirteen, I spent the summer in Kentucky with relatives. My dad was one of twelve children. Several still lived within easy traveling distance of the original homestead, a farm in a small place named Lost Creek just a few miles from Winchester, the town where I was born. I loved being there. I divided my time between my various aunts, uncles, and cousins.

What I loved especially was all the yummy food. Every Sunday afternoon after church, at the farmhouse in Lost Creek, Grandma hosted at a long table set for at least twenty. The women invaded the kitchen with great enthusiasm. Grandma whipped up mounds of fluffy mashed potatoes, fried chicken, gravy, and baked cornbread, and attended to the already long-simmering shucky beans. Aunt Ruth sliced the just-picked tomatoes and the smoked ham from the smokehouse. Aunt Golden always brought a huge chocolate layer cake. There was a large pitcher of iced tea and a pitcher of milk that was fresh from cow to table.

When I was at Aunt Fern's, she'd make double-sized slices of gorgeous white bread into toast, slathered with butter and black cherry jelly. Just for me!

Aunt Golden also made the best banana pudding in the world. There were no admonitions about manners. No restrictions about what combined with what. Have another helping! Have another piece of cake!

I was in gustatory heaven.

As the weeks slid by, I noticed that psoriatic lesions were beginning to pop out in places other than my scalp! There they were, peeping out around the edges of my hairline. In my eyebrows. On my arms. Legs. Belly. All over my body!

That's when I started reading some of the health books Mother had left lying around. They included *You Are What You Eat* by Dr. Victor Lindlahr, and the entire set of Bernarr MacFadden's *Encyclopedia of Physical Culture.*

Mother also subscribed to the monthly journal called the *Hygienic Review* from Dr. Herbert M. Shelton. On the cover was an illustration of Hygieia, the Greek goddess of health and cleanliness, bathed in sunrays and clutching in her long graceful fingers a book with the title Truth on its cover. The subtitle of the magazine was *Let Us Have Truth though the Heavens Fall.*

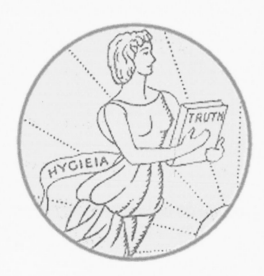

In my spotted state, I was highly motivated to seek out the truth potentially lurking in those pages.

Dr. Shelton's advice was identical to Dr. Dahl's. It included information on therapeutic fasting and eating for better health.

It was radical! But it promised hope for me. I decided there was no choice but to give it a try.

And so began my long, difficult, yet often exhilarating journey to get surcease from what has been called "the heartbreak of psoriasis." I was almost fifteen. Not too young to take it upon myself to find answers. Even though Mother had pushed it on me, she was too enmeshed in her own concerns to give me the help and comfort I needed. I couldn't begin to envision that less than two decades later, I would be a leading figure in the health movement that had been founded by Dr. Shelton; that we would be corresponding and attending the same national health conventions; and that he would publish an article I wrote in his *Hygienic Review.*

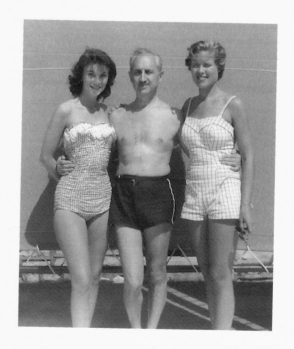

My New Life

In Victor Lindlahr's 1940 book *You Are What You Eat*, there was a chart of all major fruits and vegetables, and the vitamins and minerals each contained. At the top were the ones that were highest in everything. I studied it. I wanted to start at the top! Heading the list was curly parsley, which was loaded up with everything good. Next came kale, then collard greens, and so on.

I learned that the dark greens contain not only all the vitamins and minerals needed for super health, but also all the amino acids that are the building blocks of proteins.

And I discovered that we can make our own finished proteins from these magic elements ... just as do the animals that most people think they have to eat to get their protein.

Plus I learned that when you eat an animal to get what's called "second-hand protein," you also get the urea, uric acid, and other toxic byproducts (including cholesterol) of the animal's metabolism, which doubles the toxins your cells have to unload to keep your bloodstream at the right pH level for you to stay alive.

I kept researching over the course of a few years and found out that psoriatics' skin cells multiply thirty to forty times faster than normal. It's a benign cancer. And since protein is a building and growth nutrient, it exacerbates the manufacture of skin cells, which is where the exfoliation comes in.

I first came across the word *diathesis* in one of Dr. Shelton's articles in the *Hygienic Review*. (I always kept a dictionary handy when reading Shelton.) It means genetic predisposition. It's a flaw that's coded into cells at conception, and it's there permanently. Psoriasis was my diathesis.

I further discovered that psoriatics are predisposed to arthritis. When you have the double whammy, it's called psorioarthritis... and can be crippling.

The more I learned, the more excited I became about starting anew. So I plunged in.

The hardest part was that how I ate set me apart from my peers. I noticed that the new diet was keeping me at 120 pounds, which was nice, but it was also making me look very young for my age. I was often mistaken for thirteen or fourteen—I wasn't too happy about that!

I remember one time going with my boyfriend John and another couple for a bite to eat after a skating party. They ordered burgers and Cokes. I ordered a glass of apple juice—there was nothing on the menu I would eat. John looked my way and said, "What are you, one of them thar *vegetarians*?" I was humiliated. I wished I could have dropped through the floor. Those were the days when no one you ever knew or heard of was a vegetarian. For years I felt odd and just different from anyone else in my world. I was concerned with what people would think. But since I was more concerned that my psoriasis would pop out again, I was determined to stick to the new way of eating. I knew from my research that animal fats and excess protein were promoters of my condition.

As the years passed I read and studied more on the subject of nutrition. I completely lost any desire I ever had for flesh foods. I also began looking behind the scenes into animal food production. Philosophy became intertwined with nutrition and biochemistry in my scheme of things. I'd learned that most of the famous philosophers and great thinkers of the ages had been vegetarians. George Bernard Shaw had said, "My own objection to being carnivorous, in so far as it is not instinctive, is that it involves an enormous slavery of men to beasts as their valets, nurses, mid-wives, and slaughterers." Dr. Shelton quoted this in the second volume of his *Hygienic System, Orthotrophy*, continuing in his own words: "Man's slavery to meat animals is appalling. He lives with them in the most unhygienic conditions, in order that he may eat dead carcasses. He little dreams of the gigantic waste of human energy and food that the practice involves."

Studying great thinkers had added another dimension to my new lifestyle. I couldn't foresee, then, that one day a prominent journalist, Eric Schlosser, whose 2001 book *Fast Food Nation* became a bestseller, would autograph my copy of his book: "For Joy Gross, who knew all these things way before me. It was a pleasure meeting you."

Thinking about where what you're eating comes from may help you to avoid or give up some of the most acid-forming foods, the ones that are the most addictive—especially animal foods such as meat, eggs, and dairy products. Remind yourself that the huge industries behind these foods use whatever methods they can to enhance their products' appeal and grow their market. One way they do this is to claim nutritional benefits for their products. In this process, the "science" of nutrition becomes the "business" of marketing. They keep tabs on "dangerous" research and actively market their version, regardless of potentially dangerous health effects.

They're the ones who tell you that meat builds strong muscles and gives you strength; and that all those refined breakfast cereals give you great energy. That milk is good for you, even though milk is baby food and when you're not a baby anymore, you lose the enzyme called lactase, which digests the milk sugar lactose. Not to mention that milk is pasteurized, which makes absorbing its protein more difficult, and it contains the residues of antibiotics, hormones, and other medicines given to the cows, which can lead to allergies and other health problems.

My files contain research material I've sought out and saved for many years. I could cite instance after instance of such evidence in an attempt to encourage you to take charge of your own health, your own body, your own life. But I'll share just one of the quotes that have influenced me: "The aim of medicine is to prevent disease and prolong life; the ideal of medicine is to eliminate the need of a physician"—the words of Dr. William J. Mayo, cofounder of the Mayo Clinic.

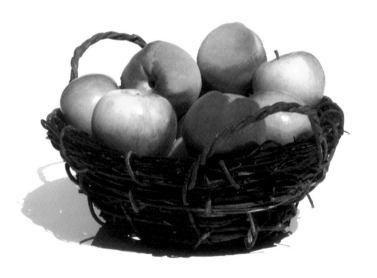

NATURE BOY

After a brief unhappy stint at Montreat College in North Carolina, I was working as a telephone operator in Asheville. Through an ad in a national newspaper, the *American Vegetarian* (precursor to the current *Vegetarian Times* magazine), I learned about a vegetarian commune in Florida that was looking for young people to do office work and other jobs in return for room and board. I was excited about the possibility of being in a sunny place, as sunlight is a temporary boon for psoriasis.

I quit my job and bought a train ticket to Sebring, Florida. The name of the place I was headed for was Lorida—a few miles south and off the beaten path of Sebring.

I arrived at an isolated small community owned and operated by a strangely interesting man who had long black hair and a stringy black beard. His name was Walter Siegmeister. He had a Ph.D. in philosophy from New York University. His brother Elie Siegmeister, I learned by noticing phonograph records stashed in his office, was a famous American composer, conductor, and author.

We were half a dozen workers. Our job was helping Siggie, as we called him, run his mail-order business selling subscriptions to his newsletter *Biosophy*, in which he touted what might now be called New Age philosophy. We lived in rustic cabins, bathed in nearby Lake Istapoga, and ate the produce from the large organic garden and the carefully tended papaya and orange trees. I reveled in the luscious tree-ripened papayas and the outdoor living style. We did our office work on a long table that was set up out in the open. My daily outfit was a two-piece bathing suit.

One of the inhabitants was a suntanned, well-muscled young man with long blond hair and a beard to match. He expounded on philosophy for hours at a time with other members of the group, and he ate a dozen oranges for breakfast every morning.

"Wow!" I thought. "A man who eats like I do!"

A few months later, we were married. I was nineteen years old.

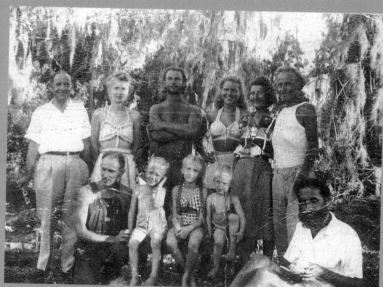

TEN YEARS LATER

Ten years and three children later, I realized that it takes more than eating oranges together for breakfast to make a marriage work.

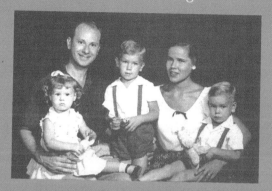

Toward the end of my marriage to Louis, while we were living in St. Louis, Missouri, the *American Vegetarian* ran a front-page lead story with photographs of my family and me. I began getting mail from all over the country, including from members of the American Natural Hygiene Society (ANHS), now the National Health Association headquartered in Tampa, Florida. I became active in the group.

In 1955, I attended my first national ANHS convention, which was held in Washington, DC, at the Shoreham Hotel. I was elected the national Secretary-Treasurer.

Back home I set up office in my five-year-old daughter Betsy's bedroom, which was handily adjacent to the kitchen. I spent many days revising lists, organizing, and sending out membership renewal notices. I took over the until-then erratically published ANHS newsletter and turned it into a sophisticated little bimonthly magazine.

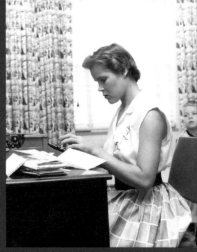

As the membership grew, I became well known for recruiting new members to the movement. Among them were C. E. Doolin, founder of the Frito-Lay Company in San Antonio, Texas; and U Thant, the first Secretary General of the United Nations, who commended me for my work.

During the summer of 1958, the annual ANHS convention was held in St. Louis, and I was the co-chairperson. Among the three hundred attendees was a black man from New York named Robert Earl Jones. The hotel management told us that he couldn't stay in that hotel. We told the management that if Robert Earl went, we would all go. Robert Earl Jones stayed. A few years later he introduced me to his son, also a stage and film actor, James Earl Jones. Robert Earl and I remained friends throughout his long life.

PAWLING HEALTH MANOR

A year after my divorce from Louis, and two days after Christmas 1958, I married Robert Gross, a physiologist from New York City who was active in the American Natural Hygiene Society.

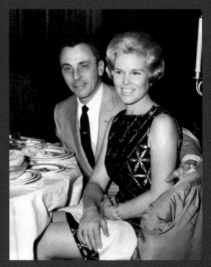

In the spring of 1959, Bob and I pooled our resources—two used cars, my three children and his one, with a total of $5,000 between us—and headed for Hyde Park, New York. We leased, with an option to buy, a historic Georgian mansion sitting atop a hill overlooking the majestic Hudson River. We all moved into the third floor, which had been servants' quarters in bygone years. We renamed the mansion the Pawling Health Manor, from its original Pawling Manor (it's now renamed the Belvedere Mansion, an event place). Our first ads were placed in the classified section of the *New York Times*.

On Memorial Day in 1959, we opened our doors. We were immediately filled to capacity. Many of my and Bob's followers became our paying guests.

Through the years of hard work, and often pain, at Pawling Health Manor, I have been privileged to share my experiences and growing knowledge with tens of thousands of people who spent time with us. I had spent so many difficult years on my own delving, studying, and experimenting with fasting, veganism, and vegetarianism in an effort to help myself. How lucky these people were, I'd think, remembering how I'd struggled so, with no health haven supervision or help. It was tremendously gratifying to witness the remarkable health improvements and miraculous recoveries happening non-stop, week in and week out, year in and year out, at the Manor.

Grateful guests spread the word and came back for refreshers. Weekly ads in the *New York Times* and later *New York Magazine* drew in lots of new guests, many of them initially interested in losing weight, and lose they did! Some of them even wrote major articles for magazines and newspapers proclaiming their happiness with results they'd received. A few wrote books about their experiences.

Ours was a strict regimen, relying on very simple, individually prescribed and served vegan meals with supervised fasting for those who qualified. Resting was a prescribed necessity for fasters. We offered gentle yoga instruction. Lectures were designed to inspire and instruct. There was a well-equipped gymnasium donated to us by a grateful long-term guest who had conquered a weight problem and serious arthritis.

In the meantime, a boxing camp was established in the vicinity. Cus D'Amato, the famous trainer who had more champions than any trainer in the world, set up headquarters there. Our family went often to watch Cus train young boxers. It was there we met José Torres, the former light heavyweight champion of the world, and Pete Hamill, the journalist, who was also a boxing enthusiast, as was Bob. Cus ended up eventually being ousted by his backer, Jimmy Iselin. Bob invited him to set up his boxing ring in our gym. When I gave my exercise classes, the ladies and I climbed over the ropes into the ring, which accommodated us very well.

Spectators from far and near came on weekends to watch Cus D'Amato train his young boxers. Pete and various of his five brothers would show up. Eventually Pete's brother Brian met my daughter Betsy. Brian soon after became my son-in-law.

A few years later I decided we needed the gym space for our Manor guests. And so it was that I told Cus he'd have to find another home for his boxing ring. He set up in a gym in Catskill, just across the river and north a bit. It was there, while teaching kids from a facility for troubled boys, that Cus discovered another fighter—future heavyweight champion Mike Tyson (now a vegan!).

CHIEF COOK AND BOTTLE-WASHER

From the beginning of Pawling Health Manor, I was the chief kitchen person as well as the shopper and overall housekeeping supervisor—a huge job considering I also had three small children and later, two additional ones.

Besides my other jobs I trained kitchen staff in how to make beautiful nutritious salads, steam vegetables, make the magic Green Goddess chlorophyll-rich juice, and put together luscious fruit plates.

I gave talks several times a week on nutrition, vegetarianism, and healthy food preparation. A gorgeous, delicious vegetarian food demonstration and luncheon on Saturdays, going-home day for most, celebrated the departing guests' weight loss and improved health.

Although Bob and I didn't succeed in our marriage, we were crucial to each other in many ways. I learned infinitely more about the basic principles of physiology and nutrition from him.

One of our daughters, Debbie, has for years been a news anchor at WCBS Radio. And another daughter, Wendy, a former psychotherapist, is Managing Director of Town Real Estate in New York City and in 2006 was designated by the *New York Post* as one of New York City's fifty most powerful women. My daughter Betsy is now a celebrated Hudson Valley artist. She owns a studio in nearby Red Hook where her many students come to learn her secrets. My son David opened the very first health foods store in the vicinity as well as a popular restaurant. Louie, another son, was for over forty years a valued staff member at our local hospital, now retired. So Bob and I got a lot of things right.

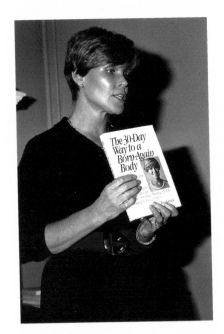

BEING A STAR

We had many luminous celebrities stay at Pawling. One of our earliest and most memorable guests was Veronica Lake, the sultry beauty whose waterfall of blonde locks was styled to obscure half her face. Veronica was the star of hit Hollywood movies in the 1940s and a favorite pin-up girl for the GIs overseas in World War II.

Veronica came with her friend Nat Perlow, hardboiled editor of the *Police Gazette*. Veronica was a smoker, and smoking wasn't permitted at the Manor. So every evening the two of them hightailed it to the nearby town of Rhinebeck and ate at the bar of Foster's Coach House Tavern.

Although Veronica was on crutches due to a leg injury and her famous peek-a-boo hair was pulled snugly back into a ponytail, she was quickly recognized as she lit up and downed her vodkas.

But most of our clients followed our regime.

Throughout the thirty-plus years of work at the Manor, I continued to live by the same health principles that led me there. I realized more than ever that these principles had not only allowed me to keep my psoriasis under control, but had also kept me healthy and drug- and physician-free through menopause, the stress of running the Manor, raising children, and sharing my energy in the counseling of our tens of thousands of guests.

Most men and women my age are old-looking. They have degenerative diseases such as arthritis, obesity, liver and gallbladder problems, heart problems, and cancer. They're dependent on "meds" to get through. And they undergo all kinds of surgeries to stay alive.

I take no medicines and no supplements. I don't need a doctor, am involved in numerous local causes, take courses at nearby Bard College, play bridge, paint and create art ... and still am attractive to the opposite sex!

I spend precious time with my five grandchildren, who range in age from nine to twenty-nine. My first great-granddaughter, Seychelle, is our fourth-generation vegetarian.

Recently I received a Facebook message from my granddaughter Cara's cousin Katie, in response to some photos Cara had posted. I'd like to share her message with you:

"Joy! You're amazing and beautiful! Your dedication and commitment to a healthy lifestyle is a real inspiration to me. I can only hope that I am half as hot and healthy as you when I'm lucky enough to be a grandma!"

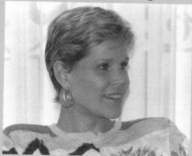 You too can be hot and healthy—and have the vitality of a star—at any age.

Keep reading!

YOU ARE YOUR CELLS

For over three decades at Pawling Health Manor, I watched more than 60,000 people turn their lives from unhealthy, low-energy states of sterile existence into robust, exciting, pleasure-packed adventures.

And I saw people who were continually drained by chronic low-grade illnesses free themselves from sickness to become beautiful and whole.

They learned that to "go on a diet" is a superficial approach to health and beauty—most people begin thinking right away, "When can I get off this no-fun diet?" They learned that there's no miraculous pill or vitamin, no magical drink that will bring lasting results.

True health is wholeness. It's having everything—mind, body, and soul—in a beautiful state of balance. To get to that state you must learn how to nourish your body the way nature intended it to be nourished. This means, in great part, learning how to eat differently.

What you put into your body has an immediate effect; it makes a difference in how you look, how you feel, how quickly you age, and how long you will live.

By changing to a new way of eating and thinking—by making it easier for your ever-faithful and hardworking cells to do their job—you can change your body and your world.

CELL TALK

"Cells are obedient and noble, perpetually hardworking, devoted to the health and survival of the organism they form," wrote cytologist L. L. Larison Cudmore in her book *The Center of Life: A Natural History of the Cell*.

There's an exciting drama that goes on inside you. It's the story of your cells, and the acid–alkaline, or pH, balance of your bloodstream, which has to be maintained at a precise level for you to live.

Our bodies are composed of more than fifty trillion cells, all working together as an organism for the survival and wellbeing of the whole you!

In order to do this, though, their needs must be met. Our cells require:

Sunlight
Oxygen
Water
Food
Excretion
Rest

The first three are straightforward. However, I'm going to give you a different perspective on what food, excretion, and rest mean as they relate to your cells.

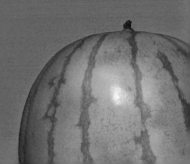

FOOD

What is food, exactly? Is it anything you eat? Not really. Food is only that which can be converted into functioning tissue.

For example, what we call "junk food" is really just junk, because it can't be converted into functioning tissue. The same goes for alcohol, caffeine, tea, chocolate, spices, cereal products made from refined sugars and flours, saturated fats, vinegar, soft drinks, and the acids in the animal foods you eat: beef, pork, poultry, fish, and seafood. (Those acids are the poisonous by-products of the animals' metabolism, such as urea and uric acid.)

These "foods" can't be used by your cells. On the contrary, they clog up the works. What your cells can't use becomes a poison, or toxin, that has to be removed so it doesn't upset the acid to alkaline (pH) balance of your bloodstream—which, in order for you to live, must be maintained at a constant 80 percent alkaline to 20 percent acid ratio.

In his book *The pH Miracle: Balance Your Diet, Reclaim Your Health*, physiologist Dr. Robert O. Young explains it this way: "The pH level of our internal fluids affects every cell in our bodies. The entire metabolic process depends on an alkaline environment. Chronic over-acidity corrodes body tissue, and if left unchecked will interrupt all cellular activities and functions, from the beating of your heart to the neural firing of your brain. In other words, over-acidity interferes with life itself. It is at the root of all sickness and disease. … It is also what keeps you fat."

So acid "stuff" you overeat becomes, in essence, garbage in your system. It becomes a threat to the survival of your cells—which are you! And that brings us to our next topic.

EXCRETION

The residues left in your system that threaten that integrity of your pH are called "ash"—specifically, acid ash.

There's also alkaline ash, which is good, and is used to help neutralize the bad stuff. It comes from the fresh fruits and veggies you eat.

Your diligent, hard-working cells have to get rid of the potentially dangerous acidic garbage. They do so by calling into action a cleanup crew called the buffer system. It's comprised of your kidneys, your lungs, and your skin. It's the water system of your body. Accumulated acid waste is excreted via your kidneys in the form of urine; your lungs by way of your breath; and your skin in the form of evaporation (armpits, crotch, feet) or as pimples, sores, or rashes. (In my case, because of my psoriatic predisposition, it was patches of psoriasis.)

An emergency helper in this detox process is your ever faithful and hardworking liver.

In desperation, your cleanup crew may deposit leftover garbage in out-of-the-way places such as your fat cells, in the form of tumors, or in your liver. During fasting these tumors are often autolyzed (broken down) and used as substitute fuel. So is your fat.

Many of our Manor guests were amazed when they not only lost weight, but saw their tumors miraculously vanish after fasting and getting their systems to a more alkaline state.

It was fascinating to see how different types of acidic garbage being eliminated made themselves evident when people were fasting. I could identify various guests' fasting breath smells. For example, Barry, a man of forty, told us he'd read about a fish diet to help lose weight. He'd eaten nothing but fish for two weeks. As he fasted, his breath started smelling like rotten fish. It became so intense you had to hold your breath to keep from gagging when you walked into the room. All that unusable acid waste from the fish was finally being eliminated from his cells.

The most opportune time for this excretion activity to happen is when you're resting, and especially when you're asleep. The next section explains why.

REST

Energy is life. The inner drama of your cells' efforts to keep you alive and well must be continually fueled by energy. The aim, remember, is to maintain that necessary pH level of your bloodstream—7.35 to 7.45. This process takes place more rapidly when you're resting and sleeping. The reason has to do with your brain and your muscles.

Your brain uses 20 to 25 percent of your body's total energy supply. When you're at rest, especially when you're asleep, power that would be used to keep your brain functioning—and, to a lesser extent, your muscles for physical activity—becomes available to help with the excretion process, sweeping out the acid toxins.

That's actually what detox refers to: getting rid of the garbage. That's one good reason why fasting or going on a juicy fruit diet for a few days is so good for you. And it's also why, when people fasted at Pawling Health Manor, Dr. Gross insisted that they rest instead of being physically active. Clients who rested invariably lost more weight than those who insisted on mixing detox with exercise.

Another great thing that happens during the fast is that as your taste buds begin to clean out, hunger disappears. You get a substitute fuel called ketone bodies—the breakdown residues from toxins such as yucky fat and dirty water—and you lose your appetite. That's ketosis. Your hardworking cells love this opportunity to houseclean. I like to think that they tell themselves and each other, "Thank heaven! Finally! We can do this job we haven't had the time or energy to do properly before! Let's hurry and see how much we can get done!"

They continue, "We know from long experience that we will soon have to get back to that first job of taking in so much more than is needed, which robs us of the extra energy we need to scrape out the sludge that is hidden away in our secret hiding places." (The liver is one of those places.) "Let's make hay while the sun shines!"

In his award-winning book *The Lives of a Cell,* Lewis Thomas writes that at the moment of conception there is coded into your cells an energy potential that determines the length of time, under ideal conditions, you will live. Thomas calls it your "genetic timetable." You gradually use up this energy potential as you live your life; and you use it up more quickly when you make your cells work harder than they should have to.

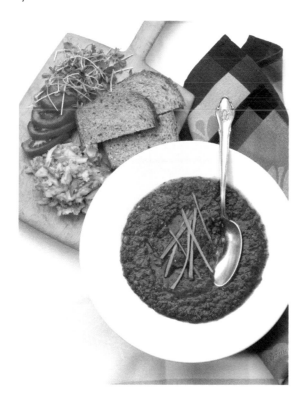

WHAT THE EXPERTS SAY

My nearly seventy-year fascination with chlorophyll, green, oxygen, pH, and Life reflects the physiological principles upon which life itself is based. One of the great pioneers in this work was Otto Warburg, M.D., who won the Nobel Prize in Medicine in 1931 for discovering that a lack of oxygen within the body leads to a pileup of acidic and fermenting dead cells and is the beginning of cancer and all disease; and that oxygen, which is found abundantly in chlorophyll, is a powerful alkalinizer. It's the magic ingredient that is necessary for life to exist. Warburg was a giant in advocating the alkaline-leaning, organic, and green diet. He lived into his nineties and ate a spartan organic alkalinizing diet.

The proof is in the pudding, as the saying goes. Dr. Warburg's discoveries prove my dietary philosophy and way of eating and living—that green growing things are loaded with oxygen, the magic ingredient that is necessary for your bloodstream to stay at the 80 percent alkaline mark, which is what keeps you living.

High heat greatly diminishes the phytonutrient content of greens, thus the importance of eating raw green leafy vegetables and drinking smoothies and green juice. (Heat over 115 degrees kills the enzymes that are the trigger mechanisms that run your body.) Warburg proved that when cells don't get the oxygen, both from breathing and from eating alkalinizing food (especially the chlorophyll-rich ones), they ferment—the cells just pile up and begin to die, right there inside of you. That fermentation process is totally acidic. If the acid ultimately invades the bloodstream itself, it is fatal. Incidentally, the pH test is the test that's done for the detection of cancer.

Dr. Caldwell B. Esselstyn Jr., M.D., says in his book *Prevent and Reverse Heart Disease*, "For most physicians, nutrition is not of significant interest. It is not a significant pillar of medical education; each generation of medical students learns about a different set of pills and procedures, but receives almost no training in disease prevention. And in practice, doctors are not rewarded for educating patients about the merits of truly healthy lifestyles."

Many other distinguished physicians and scientists have taken up Dr. Warburg's cause. For example, Joel Fuhrman, M.D., widely acclaimed as an authority in the field of nutrition and author of the bestselling 2003 book *Eat to Live* wrote, "The healthiest bodies are those with a high alkaline and low acid pH. Consuming heavy doses of chlorophyll is necessary to achieve that balance." Physiologist Robert O. Young in his book *The pH Miracle* explains it this way: "The pH level of our internal fluids affects every cell in our bodies. The entire metabolic process depends on an alkaline environment. Chronic over-acidity corrodes body tissue, and if left unchecked will interrupt all cellular activities and functions—in other words, over-acidity interferes

with life itself. It is at the root of all sickness and disease."

Dr. Amy Joy Lanou, Professor of Health and Wellness at the University of North Carolina at Asheville, is the author of a 2009 book *Building Bone Vitality*. Regarding the notion that animal foods are necessary for bone health, she wrote: "The low-acid theory is finally emerging from the refined confines of research laboratories into the practice of medicine. ... The low-acid theory is gaining momentum. Research increasingly supports a plant-based diet for bone health. ... Many scientists who not long ago dismissed the low-acid theory have changed their minds."

R. Keith McCormick, a chiropractic physician in private practice in western Massachusetts, specializes in nutritional management of bone fragility. Here's what he has to say: "When your body is acidic, you lose more calcium through your urine, and consequently your bones' osteoclastic activity accelerates. By alkalinizing your body, you will reduce calcium loss and balance the remodeling process, which maintains the health of your skeleton."

Scientific research has shown that a lack of oxygen at the cellular level is at the very center of not only the cancer problem but the disease process in general.

Remember: Oxygen is life.

Yes, you can have an "average" lifespan if you're lucky genetically. I read the obituaries in our local newspaper every day. On average, I'd be dead by now—or most certainly on medications and worse. Well, I have no fear of those outcomes. It's what I eat and my green regimen that keeps me healthy, active, and looking younger than most people my age. My alkaline way of eating and living—and my attitude—is the secret. It is the basis for the menus and recipes I share with you in this book.

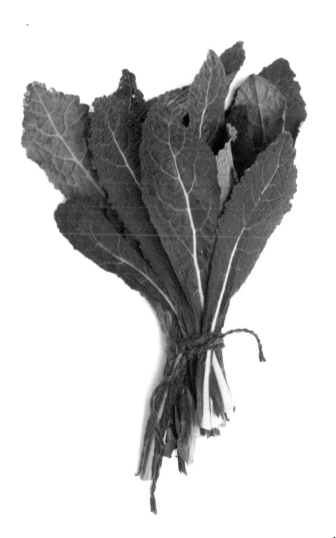

ALKALIZING AND GOING GREEN

As I explained earlier, your bloodstream must be maintained at a constant 80 percent alkaline to 20 percent acid balance for you to live. It is the job of your buffer system to make sure that the acid doesn't invade your bloodstream, and the guiding principle of your new lifelong diet will be keeping this balance in mind as you shop for food, prepare meals, and eat.

It's not always obvious which foods are acid and which are alkaline. Therefore, make use of the quick references below and make copies to carry around when shopping or eating out. Alternatively, you can download and print all the food reference lists in this chapter from my website at LiveYoungerLonger.word-press.com.

ACID

Coffee: All types, including decaffeinated.

Tea: Exceptions are green tea and herbal tea.

Meat: Beef, poultry, pork, fish, and other sea-food—anything from the body of an animal.

Eggs: All types, ranging from chicken eggs to caviar.

Dairy: Milk, yogurt, cheese, butter, and the like.

Nuts: Not as acidic as meat, eggs, and dairy, but definitely in the acid category.

Grains: Bread, pasta, rice, cereal, oats, wheat, corn (except fresh corn), and so on. The more refined the grains are, the more acidic they are.

Sweeteners: Sugar, corn syrup, and especially artificial sweeteners.

Spices: Salt, pepper, hot peppers, vinegars (except rice vinegar).

Legumes: All dried beans and peas except lentils.

Fruits: Cranberries, certain plums and prunes, and rhubarb.

Drugs: Most medications are acidic ... including antacids!

Sodas: Highly acid-forming.

ALKALINE

Fresh air: Yes, you read that right. The simple act of breathing in fresh air is alkalinizing!

Fruits: All fruits except the ones listed above. Please note that oranges, lemons, limes, grapefruits, and tomatoes are not acid-inducing in your body! They contain citric acid, which becomes highly alkalinizing when processed by your system.

Seeds: If a "nut" will sprout, it's actually a seed and not acidic. Almonds and filberts fall into this category.

Vegetables: All fresh vegetables, especially the green ones such as broccoli, collard greens, green beans, green peas, kale, mustard greens, parsley, spinach, and Swiss chard.

Let me expand upon that last point about green vegetables.

GREEN IS MAGIC.

Green plants supply the energy needs of all living things. Chlorophyll, the green coloring matter of plants, corresponds with the hemoglobin, or red coloring matter, of blood. And it's the green that ultimately makes the red.

Chloroplasts in green plants correspond to the globulin (red blood cells) in blood. It's from the globulin in our blood that we get the iron that keeps us from becoming anemic.

Chlorophyll is liquid sunlight. The chlorophyll molecule is most similar to human blood. Memorize this line. I hope it will inspire you to eat more green!

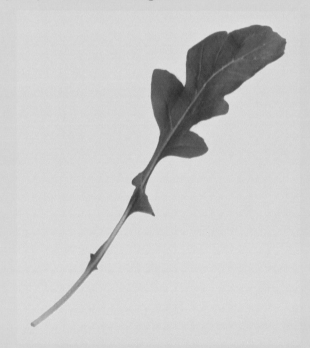

My Journey Into Green

At the age of fourteen I started learning about food values and chlorophyll from Dr. Victor Lindlahr's book *You Are What You Eat*. That's when I started making green juice for myself.

I hauled out my mother's meat grinder and ran parsley and celery through it. After the grinding I squeezed out the juice through cheesecloth. I'd drink it immediately, as I'd learned that vitamins are air-soluble and the juice had to be consumed quickly.

I noticed that when I drank the green juice, or even ate lots of green veggies, my complexion glowed. So I'd make sure to get my green fix before going square dancing with my boyfriend.

By the way, Dr. Lindlahr's groundbreaking book is now out of print (although used copies can be found through online booksellers). But some excellent recent books worth your time—that is, besides the one you're currently reading—are *Eat to Live: The Revolutionary Formula for Fast and Sustained Weight Loss* by Joel Fuhrman, M.D., with a foreword by Dr. Mehmet Oz, and *The pH Miracle: Balance Your Diet, Reclaim Your Health* by Robert O. Young, Ph.D., and Shelley Redford Young.

When I was older I bought myself a Champion juice machine. It's one of the best purchases I've ever made; and after thirty years of frequent use, it still works flawlessly! I highly recommend this product line, which debuted in 1955 and has been continually improved upon ever since. It's the only juicer I know of that can produce fresh fruit ice cream and sorbets. Champion juicers are exceptionally easy to use and clean, and—as my own experience demonstrates—super-reliable.

And yes, my juice ingredients are still parsley and celery, although I now include kale and a carrot or two. You can't improve on perfection.

BABY IN GREEN

When I was pregnant at age thirty-six with the last of my daughters, Wendy, I made a special effort to include green juice in my diet at least two or three times a week.

And after Wendy was born, I gave her a small amount of carrot and parsley juice from a bottle daily.

All five of my children are strong and healthy. Debbie and Betsy, along with Wendy, were always at the top of the class in gymnastics, and David was a soccer star.

However, from an early age, Wendy seemed to have super-strength. And she still does. She can lift and lug around objects that other women (except maybe weightlifters) can't budge.

I can't promise you the same results; but you might try my green juice regimen during your own pregnancy and for your baby afterward. It could prove handy later on whenever you need to move furniture.

HEALING IN GREEN

Back in 1980, right after a photo session for the cover of my book *The 30-Day Way to a Born-Again Body*, I started driving to see a friend who was hospitalized. On the way, a family of skunks ran out in front of my car. I swerved to avoid hitting them and lost control, smashing into a huge boulder. The accident totaled the car and landed me in the hospital with severe injuries.

After five hours of surgery, I was hospitalized for a month. However, I never ate anything from the hospital trays. The staff from the Manor brought me green juice, orange juice, salads, and fresh fruit.

When I returned home, with casts on both legs, I continued the same eating regime.

My doctors were worried about my being a vegetarian. "How are we going to get protein into you?" they asked repeatedly.

But as the months went by, periodic x-rays showed the severed and split femur, broken ankle, fractured pelvis and ribs, and smashed knee all to be healing!

I graduated from wheelchair to walker to crutches to cane—and finally was able to get back on my own two feet. And this healing occurred on a totally vegetarian, and mostly vegan, diet that included green juice.

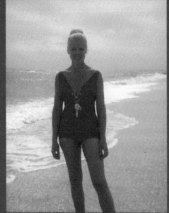

What also helped was faithfully performing water and stretching exercises. After thirty years, in addition to staying physically active, I still perform these exercises daily.

MENOPAUSE IN GREEN

If you're a woman, menopause is a time in your life when you have to deal with a biological rationale that says since you can no longer reproduce, you are no longer indispensable in nature's scheme of things. Your inner machinery slacks its vigilance in keeping you as healthy and sexy as before. It also burdens you with hot flashes and night sweats, weight gain, and your skin not glowing as it once did. You generally have to work harder to stay attractive and well.

One of the odd things that happened to me was that my breasts grew larger. I'd always been a perfect 36B. Then I crept up to a C. That was okay. But as the years went by I enlarged to a 38D, which wasn't okay. I was uncomfortable.

"Enough!" I said to those crazy cells that were having a ball proliferating in my chest. I decided to have a breast reduction.

The day after the surgery, Dr. Hagerty came into the room to check me out. This is what he said: "You have beautiful blood!"

I'd been drinking my green juice daily and faithfully. His comment was a verification of my research relating to chlorophyll and human blood. "Green makes red" is true!

And in three days I was back to my daily routine—driving, gardening, traveling, and seeing friends. It felt great to be back to my good old 36C and to recover from surgery that quickly.

What Dr. Hagerty said was proof for me that:

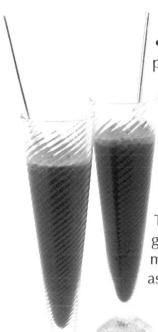

- Green is magic.

- Green juice is a big plus for me.

- Greens make my cells happy.

- A green salad a day is helping me to live younger longer.

Thinking and eating green can be just as much of a plus for you as it has been for me.

GREEN SUCCULENTS

When you first think of green succulents, you might envision munching on prickly pear cactus or harvesting the hens-and-chicks from your rock garden. Although the prickly pear cactus is indeed edible, other kinds of green succulents are much more familiar and close at hand. These plants are high in water content. And I strongly recommend that you include them in your meals as often as possible.

Green succulents are especially important. They provide water, vitamins, minerals, and amino acids (the building blocks of protein), as well as the dietary fiber you need for optimal digestion. Some people try to keep a normal pH balance by taking supplements. While this certainly is better than eating French fries as your vegetable, eating fresh greens is thousands of times better, because supplements are highly processed food and their nutritional content is altered.

These are the green succulents:

- Asparagus

- Broccoli

- Brussels sprouts

- Cauliflower

- Celery

- Collard greens

- Eggplant

- Green beans

- Kale

- Lettuce (all green varieties)
- Parsley
- Peppers
- Spinach
- Summer squash
- Swiss chard
- Turnip greens
- Turnips
- Watercress

If you choose to eat these green succulents more often than not, your body will thank you ... and reward you with health and vitality.

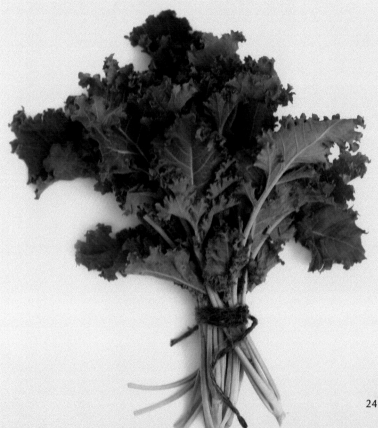

CHOOSING PRIME FRUITS AND VEGETABLES

Knowing how to choose prime fruits and vegetables, especially fruits, is crucial. Let's start with fruit. Almost all fruit is picked long before it has reached its peak of ripeness and flavor. That's not as likely to be the case if you can get locally grown, and preferably organic, produce. I live in Rhinebeck, New York, where in summer we have delicious sweet peaches, pears, plums, berries, and melons that are not picked unripe, as imported produce is. I shop at the weekly farmers' market. If you live in a city, look for sidewalk produce stands. Usually they are supplied by farms in outlying rural areas and are trucked in fresh daily.

Bananas should be at least pale yellow; store them in a dark place for a few days until they turn deep yellow with a few specks. That's when their starch has turned to sugar and they are sweet and delicious.

I adore mangos; however, they are picked green for shipping. I never buy them unless they give at least a little when pressed. Then I put them in my kitchen windowsill, often for as long as a week, until they show beautiful reds and yellows and feel soft under pressure from my fingers. I recently served a crystal bowl of sliced mangos and peaches at a bridge luncheon at my home. My lady friends were incredulous at how delicious they were. That's because they'd been ripening in the windowsill for well over a week.

yellow. If a petal can be pulled out of the top easily, it's likely to be sweet and juicy.

I don't usually buy citrus fruit during the summer months; their prime season begins in November. My favorite variety of oranges is the Florida Honeybell. I order them by the case and use them as the mainstay of my winter fruits, along with grapefruits.

Honeydew melons should be a chalky white, not greenish white. Press on the end opposite the stem end. If it gives at least a little to pressure, it will most likely be succulent and sweet. Otherwise you may be stuck with one that tastes more like a cucumber than a luscious treat. Cantaloupes should be deep yellow and have a beautiful aroma.

I concentrate more on the leafy vegetables than the ones that need cooking. Romaine lettuce and dark green lettuces, such as Boston, and arugula, Swiss chard, and kale (preferably the Lacinato variety) are my favorites. I use kale in my green juice and smoothies. I also incorporate thinly sliced kale into my tossed salads. California carrots are the sweetest and best. I use usually one medium-sized one in my green juice; otherwise I grate them for use in salad. Sprouts of any kind make a wonderful addition to any salad.

Most supermarkets today have a gorgeous and varied array of all the fresh fruits and vegetables, many of which are organic. I do a good amount of shopping in my health food store, where they have organic lacinato kale, which is difficult if not impossible to find in most other markets. I like it because it is a dark blue-green, the kind with the most potent chlorophyll content. I buy at least four bunches at a time of the darkest green parsley available, often as many as six bunches at once. I store them in airtight storage bags and use at least one bunch a day, sometimes more—one bunch for juice, one for each batch of smoothie.

Most of my meals are uncooked; it's an easier way to eat and, if you have a normal, healthy digestive system, it's healthier, since high heat destroys vitamins and enzymes. Vegetables can be lightly steamed in a small amount of water and covered with a tight-fitting lid to prevent the loss of vitamins, which are water-soluble. (It's best not to use aluminum cookware; it's porous and can contaminate your food. Stainless steel is preferable.) Potatoes and grains obviously must be cooked to render them more digestible. The exception is sprouted grains.

I use whole grains and store them in the freezer unless I can use them within a month or so, as they are susceptible to getting rancid. For instance, there are several varieties of brown rice that I use regularly. There are wheat berries. There's coarsely ground corn (used for polenta). Then there's buckwheat groats, also known as kasha, which are not grains. Whole-wheat pasta also goes into the freezer unless you're going to use it within a short period of time.

I shop at least twice a week, sometimes more often. Yes, living on prime fresh fruits

and vegetables can be more expensive. I jus-
tify that by saving on health care costs. I take
no medications; when I'm asked who my
doctor is, my answer tends to shock people:
I don't have one. Those two factors save me
the extra money to spend on what I eat. I've
proved that at least for me, health care is self
care. It starts with what you eat!

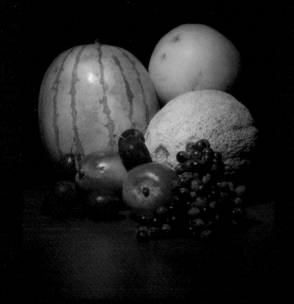

THINK ALKALINE FOR LIFE

Did you know that over-acidity may lead to
the production of more fat cells?

Fat cells provide storage for the excess garbage that your disposer cells have a hard time
removing. It's more work for your buffer system, creating another step toward early aging
and disease.

And it makes you, and millions of others,
gain fat.

The United States has the second-worst life
expectancy rate in the industrialized world.
Cancer, heart disease (including strokes), and
diabetes are the leading causes of death.

All these illnesses are closely connected
to how we eat.

Do yourself an enormous favor and start
thinking alkaline. You'll slow your aging process, increase energy, lower your risk of ill-
ness ... and get skinnier in the bargain.

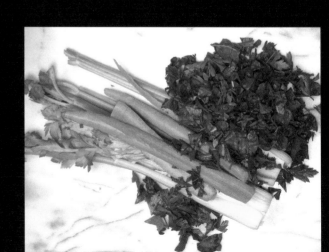

EATING OUT

I live alone. This can make it easier to eat in a simple and healthfully positive way. However, when I've had it with the solo routine and can't quickly enlist a friend, I hit the highway—Route 9, which is a ten-mile jaunt from where I live into the village of Rhinebeck. I usually decide en route which of my favorite places to visit.

And I guess you could call me an octogenarian barhopper. I've met some fascinating other loners at carefully chosen bars. For example, my last live-in relationship began at the bar of a charming French restaurant in Rhinebeck, Le Petit Bistro—almost twenty years ago. A distinguished-looking older gentleman, alone at the quaint little bar with his *Wall Street Journal* and a glass of Chardonnay, noticed me as I left my solitary corner table. He got my name, I later learned, from the bistro owner, an adorable French lady named Yvonne who was also a friend of mine. He then looked me up in the local phone directory—and the result was a happy relationship that lasted for sixteen years.

Ben wasn't by any means a follower of my health and eating philosophy, but we compromised. In my home, we ate mostly my way. He got his meat fixes during business hours, when lunching out, and the couple of times a week when we went out to dinner. I prepared some things for him that I mostly didn't eat—fresh breads, and desserts here and there. He greatly enjoyed many of the special vegetable dishes I made. And he made fresh juice for *me* every morning! His health improved during his time with me. For instance, the gout he'd suffered with for years entirely disappeared. He lived to the good age of eighty-seven. Present at the farewell service for him was Yvonne, our friend from the Bistro.

I still go to Le Petit Bistro. Although its menu leans heavily on meat and seafood, the current owner/chef Joseph Dalu is accomplished with gourmet vegetable soups (no meat stock!). And there are always beautifully prepared vegetable side dishes, which make a perfect meal for me.

Gigi Trattoria (owner/chef Laura Pensiero) in Rhinebeck has the best arugula (rughetta)

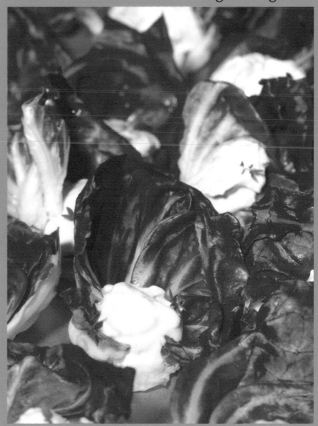

salad ever, and several other veggie selections, including whole-wheat pasta. The salad alone easily makes for a meal.

A funky spot in the adjacent town of Red Hook, the Mercato Osteria (owner/chef Franceso Buitoni) offers a fabulous kale salad. The recipe is in this book. The bartender there isn't surprised when I order a double salad. And oh, the fascinating people—many from nearby Bard College—that I've met at its friendly bar!

Other local restaurants are worthy of attention. A new eclectic jazz joint, Zen Dog Café serves a great carrot soup made with coconut milk, and Arielle, a French/Mediterranean restaurant, has a variety of interesting veggie dishes.

No matter what neighborhood you're in, you can probably find a place that offers a tasty salad or nourishing vegetable dish— even if such choices are buried in the menu or require you to make a special request for them.

CHANGING GEARS

Changing gears is all about breaking an addiction—in this case, to refined and processed starches, sugars, animal proteins, caffeine, chocolate, alcohol, and other acid-inducing foods. After a few days your cells will thank you for making their job easier. They'll now be saying, "More of the good stuff, please!" and you (you are your cells, remember!) will look forward to juicy fruits, melons, and the alkalinizing foods: the almonds, pine nuts, creamy delicious green smoothies, and luscious veggies, fruits, and salads.

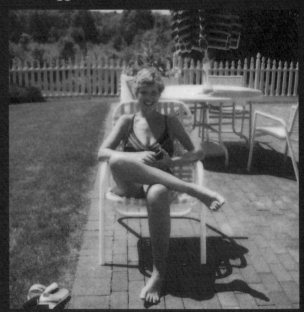

If you feel you need a hot drink to start your day, I recommend red raspberry tea with a little fresh lemon juice and real maple syrup for sweetener. (Maple syrup is unadulterated and isn't acid-forming.) By the way, before breakfast is a good time to do some stretching and deep breathing exercises. And it's alkalinizing! Try to incorporate more physical activity into your daily routine. I climb stairs, do yard work, and take a brisk walk, in addition to my early morning stretching, deep breathing, and isometrics.

My search for health was influenced and inspired by those pioneers in the field of science and medicine that I mentioned earlier in this book. I owe my vitality, wellbeing, and freedom from the traditional "old age" diseases to them and to the many other health advocates who broke ranks with tradition to become my sources of knowledge. I hope that you too may "catch" some of my enthusiasm—that it may inspire you to get on the path to eating and living alkaline and green. It will also help to alleviate the suffering of all the animals being slaughtered every day for society to keep its addictions to meat and dairy going.

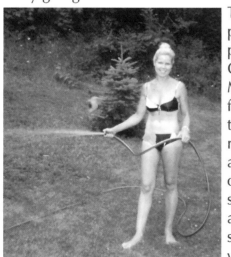
These recipes are all plant-based. Give it a try. My hope for you is that it will raise you to a new level of consciousness and a new sense of wellbeing.

TIPS FOR THE "LIVE YOUNGER... LONGER" EATING PLAN

Although becoming a vegetarian or a vegan is a great step to take (for you, for the animals, and for the planet), there's a further step to go. You can eat a lot of junk and unhealthy items and still be either a vegetarian or a vegan. You can be fat and unwell and be one of them. With that in mind, here are eight suggestions for reaching your health and weight goals. It's my own self-advice that I live by.

1. My motto is "self care." Because of my self-knowledge and my practicing of what I know as best I can, I have no fear of some mysterious disease "attacking" me. At age (almost) eighty-three, I can say to myself, "So far so good."

2. If it has eyes and moves, I don't eat it. The last time I ate a serving of animal was sixty-eight years ago.

3. I rarely eat more than I need just because it tastes good. The high water content of my food (fresh fruits and veggies) fills me and satisfies me so completely that I have a hard time taking in more calories than I need. An added benefit is that I am never thirsty. I rarely drink water.

4. I avoid processed starches and sugars.

5. I'm careful how I combine my foods. For instance, I don't eat starches with citrus fruit or starches with concentrated sugary things. That can easily lead to indigestion and gas.

6. I know which foods are either acid-inducing or alkaline-inducing inside of me and deliberately choose predominantly from the alkaline-forming group.

7. I think and eat green every day. I know that green makes red—red for blood high in iron. I sporadically do a litmus pH test, which generally shows 7.0 or a little higher. The average person's is 6.0 or less. A pH level of 7.2 is just about perfect.

8. A constant reminder for me is this quote from Ronald J. Glasser, M.D., a bestselling author and cancer expert whose book *The Greatest Battle*, linking cancer to environmental poisons, has been in my library for nearly thirty-five years: "The only real answer for disease is prevention."

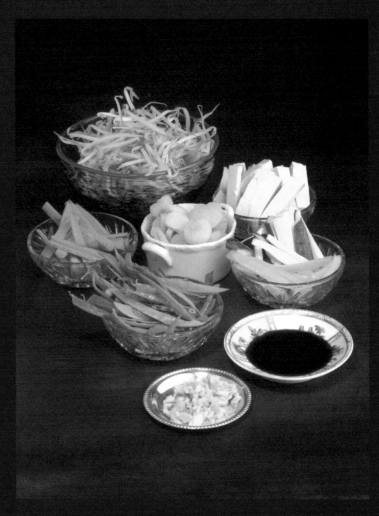

Let's Get Started

MENU SUGGESTIONS

The recipes that follow are some of my favorites. Because salt is acid-inducing and hydroscopic—it holds water and creates bloating of body tissues—I have used it sparingly in these recipes. The more simply you eat, the less the salt will be missed.

I realize that these menus may seem a little austere. However, once you've stuck to the program for a month or two and have accustomed yourself to not feeling stuffed, your body will make you feel the wisdom of it, and you'll adjust ... with increased energy and vitality.

Remind yourself that our ancestors didn't throw together all the different concoctions we do. We were designed to eat simply. Accept that ... and enjoy saying good-bye to bloating, gas, and heartburn. Not to mention those extra few pounds.

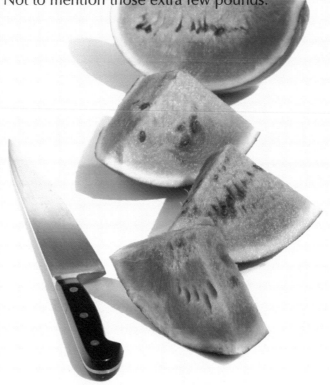

BREAKFASTS

8 ounces Green Smoothie
2 cups of honeydew melon chunks
sprinkled with blueberries
25 or 30 almonds

8 ounces Green Smoothie
½ cantaloupe filled with raspberries
¼ cup pine nuts

8 ounces Green Smoothie
generous wedge of watermelon
25 or 30 almonds

8 ounces fresh orange juice
½ honeydew melon filled with blueberries
¼ cup lightly toasted pumpkin seeds

8 ounces Green Smoothie
2 cups of watermelon chunks sprinkled with blackberries
25 or 30 almonds

8 ounces fresh grapefruit juice
2 cups cantaloupe chunks
sprinkled with strawberries
¼ cup pine nuts

8 ounces Green Smoothie
generous wedge of watermelon
¼ cup sunflower seeds

LUNCHES

1-½ cup bowl of Vegetable Soup
6 or 8 whole-wheat crackers
8 large romaine lettuce leaves
carrot and celery sticks

1-½ cup bowl of Green Pea Soup
5 or 6 rye crackers
Finger Salad

2 ripe pears cut into 4 wedges, seeded
and spread generously with homemade Cashew Butter
6 ounces of Green Smoothie

1- ½ cup Smoothie in a Bowl
1 slice of whole-wheat toast with buttery spread
5 or 6 large romaine lettuce leaves

1-½ cup bowl of steamed green lima beans with stewed tomatoes
6 ounces Green Smoothie
cucumber sticks

Avocado Treat
6 ounces Green Smoothie
6 or 8 large romaine lettuce leaves

1-½ cup bowl of tomato soup
6 whole-wheat crackers
6 ounces Green Smoothie

DINNERS

Eggplant Supreme
Steamed green peas
Squash a la Joy
Tossed Green Salad with Joy's Caesar Dressing

Potatoes Anna a la Joy
broccoli rabe
steamed carrots
Finger Salad

Luscious Linguine
steamed kale
6 or 8 large romaine lettuce leaves

Black Bean Soup
sliced beefsteak tomatoes
Arugula Salad

Carrot Ginger Soup
whole-wheat crackers
Tossed Green Salad studded with
chunks of avocado and asparagus spears

Chinese Stirfry
brown rice
Arugula Salad

Recipes listed here with capitalized titles appear in this book.

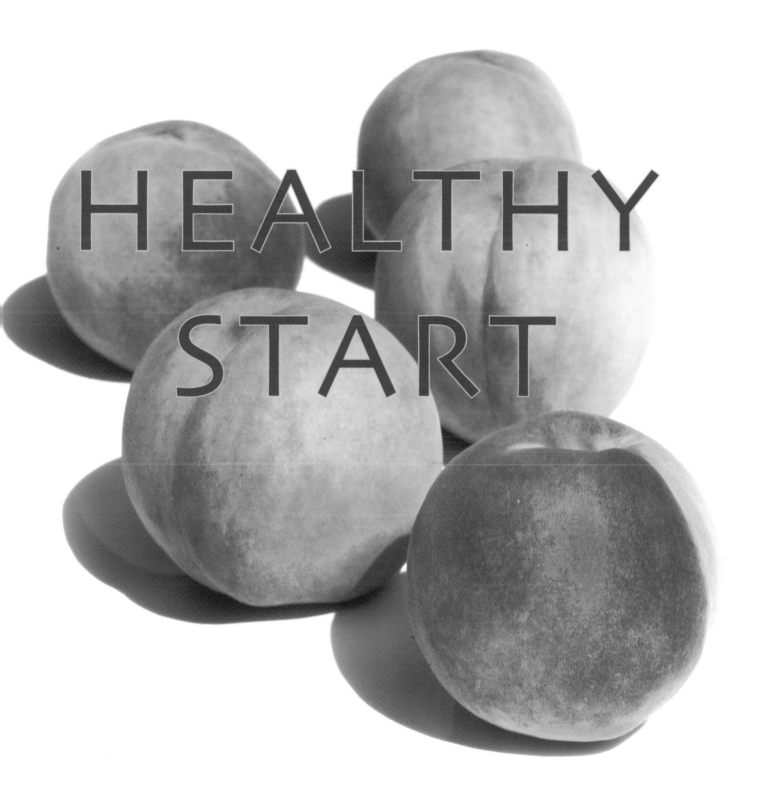

HEALTHY
START

GREEN GODDESS

Let's start with the basic recipe for Green Goddess, a blood enhancing juice I've been drinking for almost seventy years:

> 3 or 4 large crisp green celery stalks
> I medium bunch parsley
> 2 or 3 kale leaves
> 1 or 2 medium size California carrots (the sweetest kind)

Cut the stems off the parsley while it is still tied in a bunch. Chop the parsley roughly and cut the celery and carrots into chunks. Remove the stems from the kale leaves. Push the parsley through your juicer in several batches with the celery, kale, and carrot. I use a Champion Juicer, which I consider the best in terms of easy use and cleaning, although there are many other good brands available.

Drink this jade-colored, amino-acid–rich energizer immediately, because it oxidizes if you linger over it. Precious antioxidants will escape. Remind yourself as you drink that chlorophyll is more like human blood than anything that exists. It does wonders for your pH balance and puts roses in your cheeks! I try to have this blood enhancer at least four or five times a week.

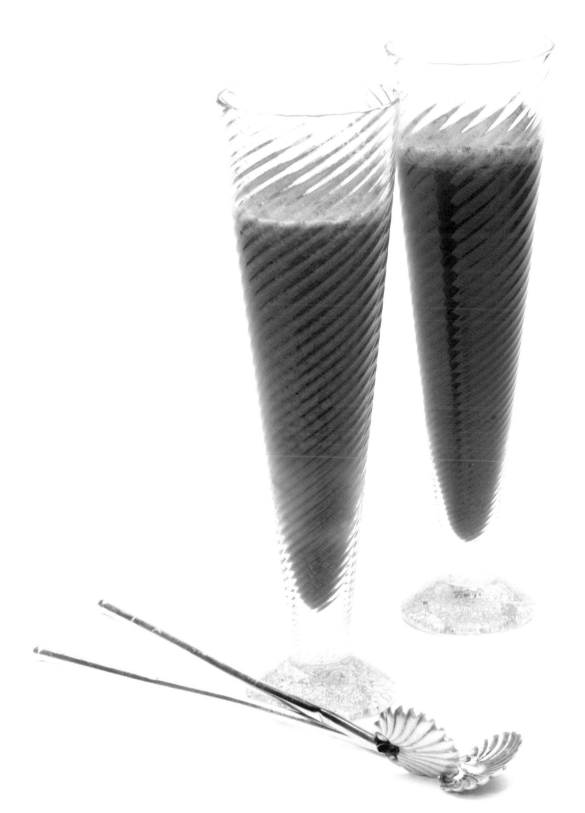

GREEN SMOOTHIE SUPREME

I love green smoothies! They taste good, give me great energy, and keep me from wanting to snack on things I shouldn't. I drink up to a quart a day. I store it in the refrigerator in a clean plastic container with a tight-fitting lid. Squirt-top plastic bottles (used for ketchup or mustard) work very well, because you can shake up the smoothie mixture and then pour it or squeeze it out through the tip into your glass. The bottles are available at any restaurant supply store.

1 medium bunch of parsley

3 or 4 kale leaves, preferably Lacinato (If you can't find Lacinato, use regular kale, or 2 leaves collard greens, or 2 cups spinach, or 2 leaves Swiss chard)

1 cup of any fresh-squeezed juice—orange, pineapple, or the like

2 tablespoons frozen apple, orange, or pineapple juice concentrate (it has no sugar or additives)

Fresh fruit, such as 2 kiwis, 2 pears, or 2 peaches and/or some grapes or a mango

Small chunk of fresh ginger root

½ lemon, including peel (remove all of the seeds)

¼ cup fresh lemon juice (which I make ahead and keep in a squirt bottle in my fridge)

About 2 tablespoons of maple syrup, or to taste, for extra sweetness if needed

Pure water as needed for proper pourability

This usually makes a quart and a half—enough for two days.

Combine all ingredients except water in the blender and process until smooth. Add water to bring it to a drinkable texture. Refrigerate.

I love my Green Smoothies and make sure there is always a covered container of the mixture in the fridge. In addition to having 8 ounces every morning with my fresh melon or citrus fruit and almonds, I have green "fixes" as needed during the day, in addition to my usual 8 ounces of pure Green Goddess Juice most days. For example, I might drink 6 ounces of Green Smoothie with lunch or have a 4-ounce "shot" mid-afternoon, and another shot before bed. I find that it keeps me energized and so satisfied that generally I don't need to eat until dinnertime. It takes away any urges for sweets or other contraband. Try it and you'll agree.

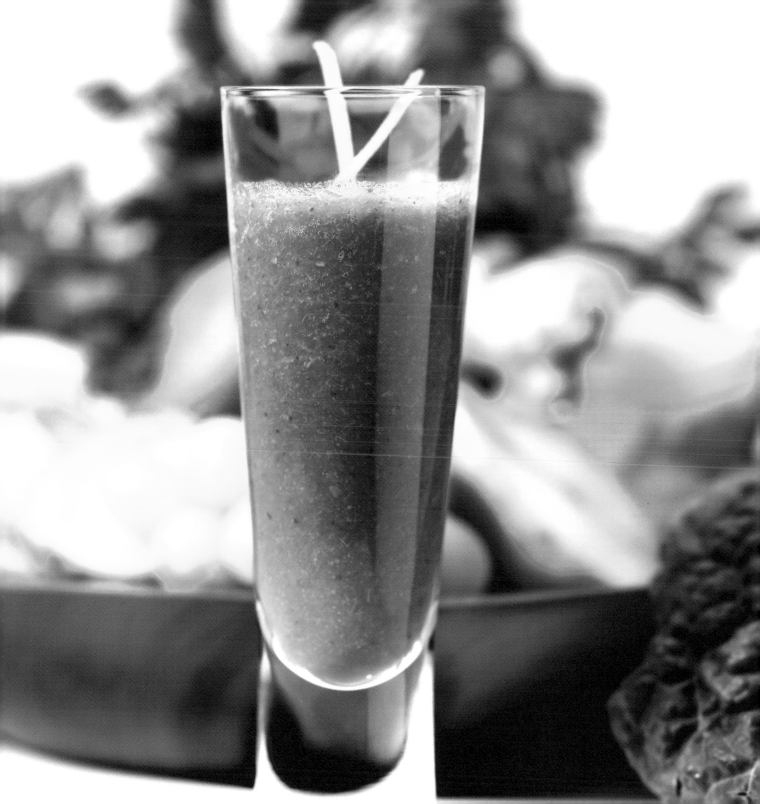

SMOOTHIE IN A BOWL

1 (15-ounce) can stewed tomatoes (preferably organic), or 1-½ cups fresh chopped tomatoes
1 medium bunch of parsley
2 or 3 leaves of kale
1 stalk of celery or 1 cucumber

Trim the stems from the parsley and the kale. Cut the celery into chunks. Peel the cucumber if desired.
Put all ingredients in a food processor or blender and process until smooth. It will be a thick mixture.
Turn out into a pretty soup bowl and eat it with a soupspoon.

This soup is so satisfying for me! I sit in a comfy spot, relax, and savor each bite. It makes a perfect lunch. If you need more to eat, add an Avocado Treat.

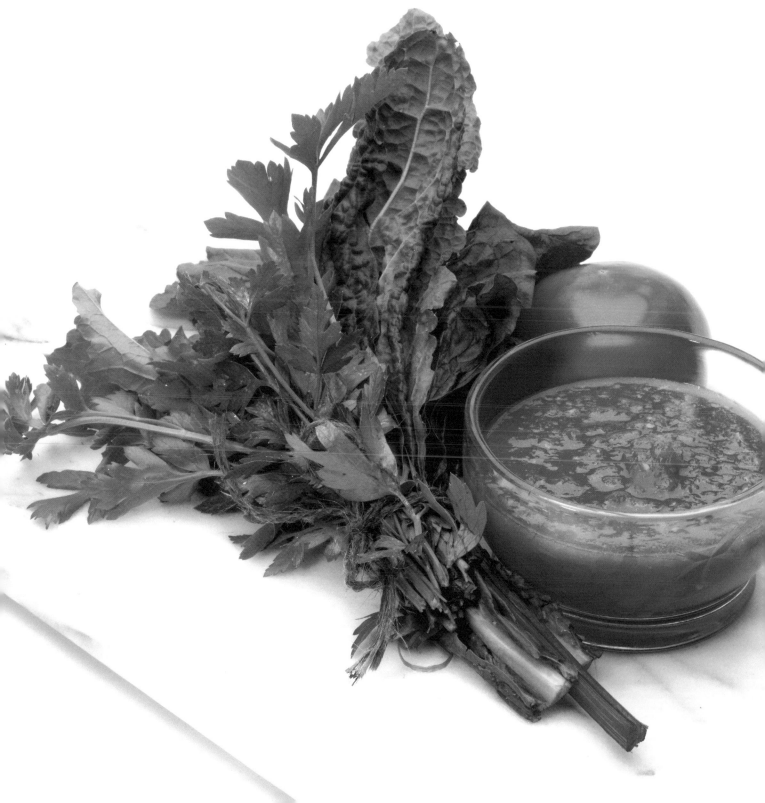

OATMEAL MY WAY

2½ cups whole oats
2 cups pure water
Pinch of sea salt (optional)
½ cup of black raisins

I make my oatmeal in electric rice steamer, although you can use a saucepan on the stove just as well. Add the water and turn the steamer to high. When the water starts to boil, turn to low, add the oats, and place lid on the steamer, and let it sit with the lid on. (As an option, add ¼ cup of raisins when you begin the process.) I just forget about it at this point and get back to it when it's convenient. The oats will have fluffed out. Alternatively, in a saucepan, bring the water to a boil and then add the oats; reduce heat to low and simmer for 25–30 minutes, stirring frequently, until soft.

At this point, with a fork, gently turn the oatmeal from the bottom—up and over— kind of an aerating process, which makes the finished dish lighter and better. A dish of this oatmeal, with a couple of tablespoons of coconut milk or Joy's Vanilla Crème (see recipe p. 103) added when serving, is a special treat. This will keep, covered, in the refrigerator for a week. I like it for a lunch, with a Green Smoothie chaser.

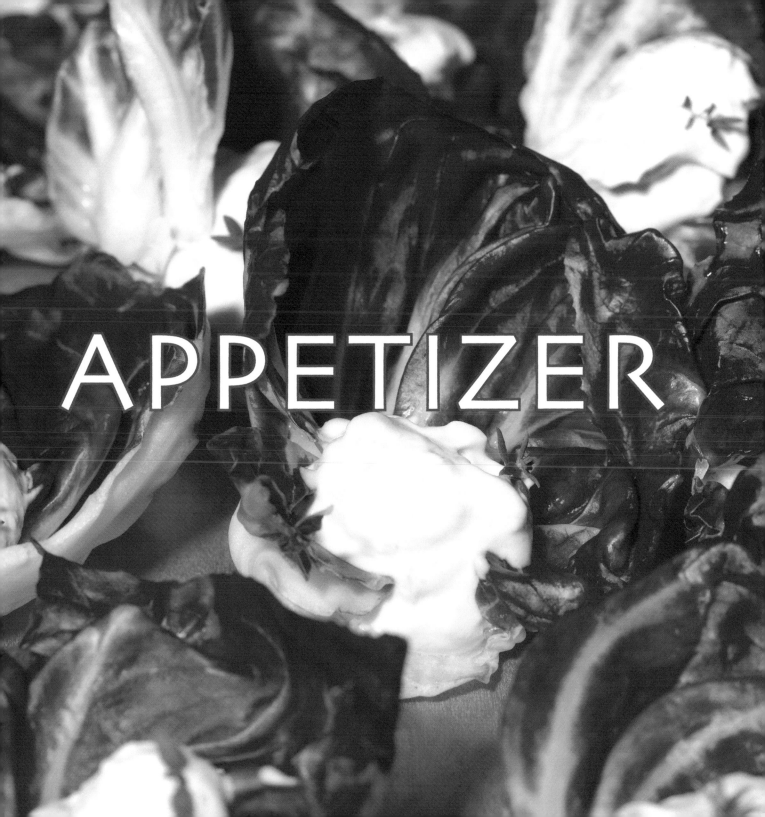

APPETIZER

STUFFED ENDIVE

1 head of Belgian endive
Joy's Tofutti Cream Cheese (see recipe p. 47)
Sprouts or watercress
Thin small carrot strips

Cut off the bottom small portion of each layer of endive as you remove the leaves, being careful not to tear the leaves. Wash carefully. Spoon a small amount of the cream cheese into the center of each leaf and garnish with the sprouts and carrot strips. Arrange on a tray and serve.

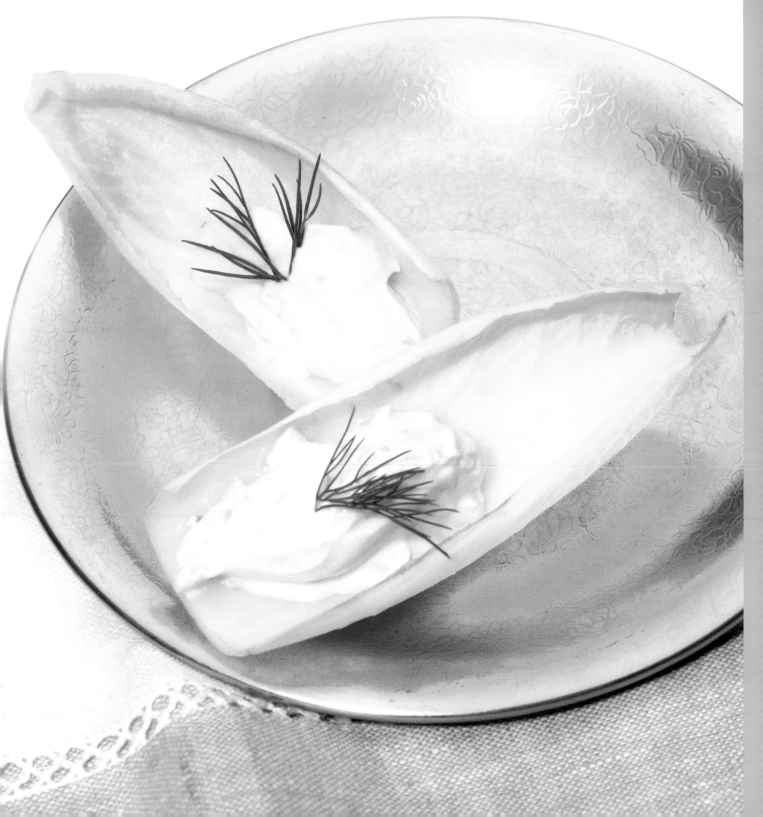

STUFFED SNOW PEAS

Select as many snow pea pods as you will need—a dozen or so, depending on how many guests you have

Joy's Tofutti Cream Cheese (see recipe p. 47)

¼ cup of chopped fresh dill, or 1 teaspoon dried dill

Green sprouts as a garnish

Red bell pepper slivers as a garnish

Incorporate the dill into the soy cream cheese.

With the sharp point of a paring knife, split the curved edge of the pea pods on the curved side. Stuff the cream cheese into each pea pod and arrange on a pretty plate or tray. Garnish with a handful of sprouts. A small sliver of red bell pepper can be inserted in the edge of each snow pea, for extra oomph.

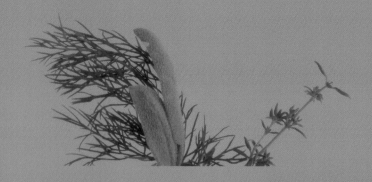

FANCY GRAPES

Medium-size bunch of grapes (seedless preferred)
½ cup almonds, finely chopped
½ cup of Joy's Tofutti Cream Cheese
Mint or grape leaves as a garnish

Joy's Tofutti Cream Cheese is simply the Tofutti-brand soy Better Than Cream Cheese to which you add your choice of herbs (maybe garlic, basil, dill, cumin, or any other in a combination that suits your taste) and a dash of fresh lemon juice. It makes the spread more interesting.

Heap the finely chopped almonds in a pile on your chopping board, next to the bowl of soy cream cheese. Roll each grape in the cream cheese, covering generously. Then carefully roll it in the chopped almonds. Repeat until all the grapes are covered.

Arrange on a pretty serving plate in the shape of a bunch of grapes; use the grape or mint leaves—or whatever other leaves are handy—for the finishing touch at the top of the bunch. These keep well in a covered container in the refrigerator and can be made ahead of time and refrigerated.

RADICCHIO NESTS

1 small head of radicchio, separated into leaves
½ cup of cashew butter
½ teaspoon of finely grated fresh ginger root
Crunchy sprouts as a garnish

For this recipe I use my own homemade cashew butter (the best!) (See Cashew Butter Balls recipe p. 95)

Lay out the small radicchio leaves. Add the ginger root to the cashew butter. Fill the center of each with a teaspoon of the cashew butter and garnish with the crunchy sprouts

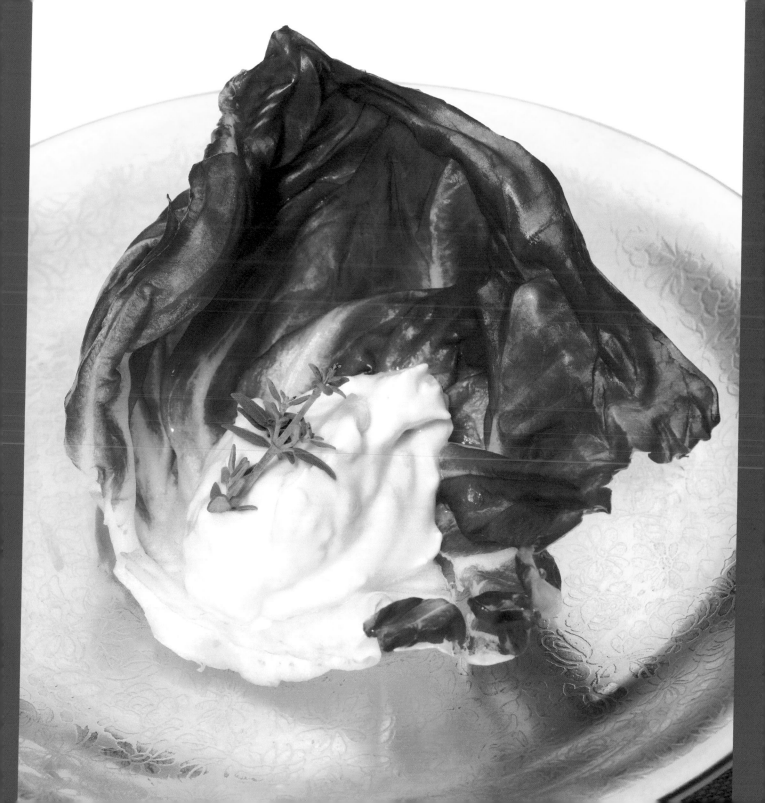

CORN CUPS FILLED WITH
CHILI BLACK BEANS

6 tablespoons non-dairy (vegan) unsalted butter at room temperature

3 ounces Tofutti Better Than Cream Cheese

1 cup unbleached flour

½ cup polenta corn meal (coarse ground)

Pinch of sea salt or other vegetable seasoning

About 1-½ cups of Yummy Chili, leftover or made fresh, with black beans

Green peas as a garnish

Preheat oven to 375 degrees.

Put all ingredients (except Yummy Chili and green peas) in food processor or standing mixer and process until it turns into a cohesive dough ball. Turn out onto a floured board, roll to ¼ -inch thickness, and cut rounds to press into small muffin tins or—my choice—a madeleine mold pan.

Bake at 375 degrees for 10 minutes, or until light golden. Remove from pan. When cool, fill centers with Yummy Chili made with black beans (see recipe p. 73). Top each cup with two or three green peas, fresh or frozen (thawed).

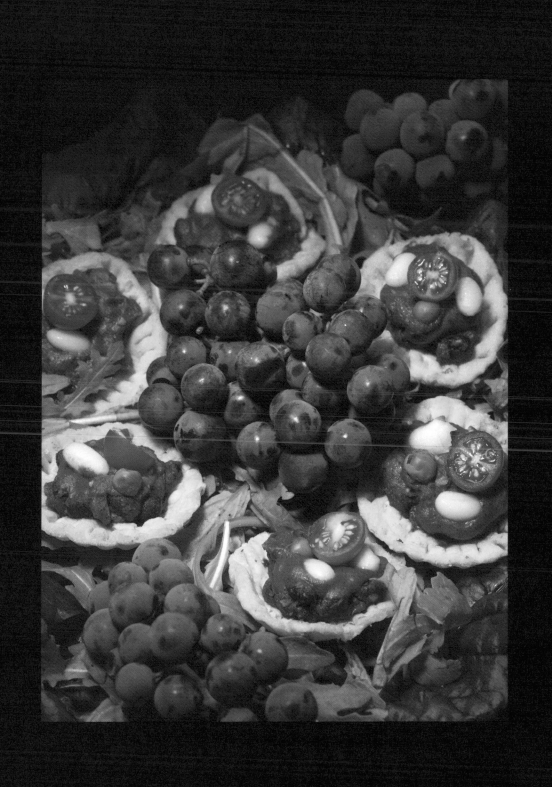

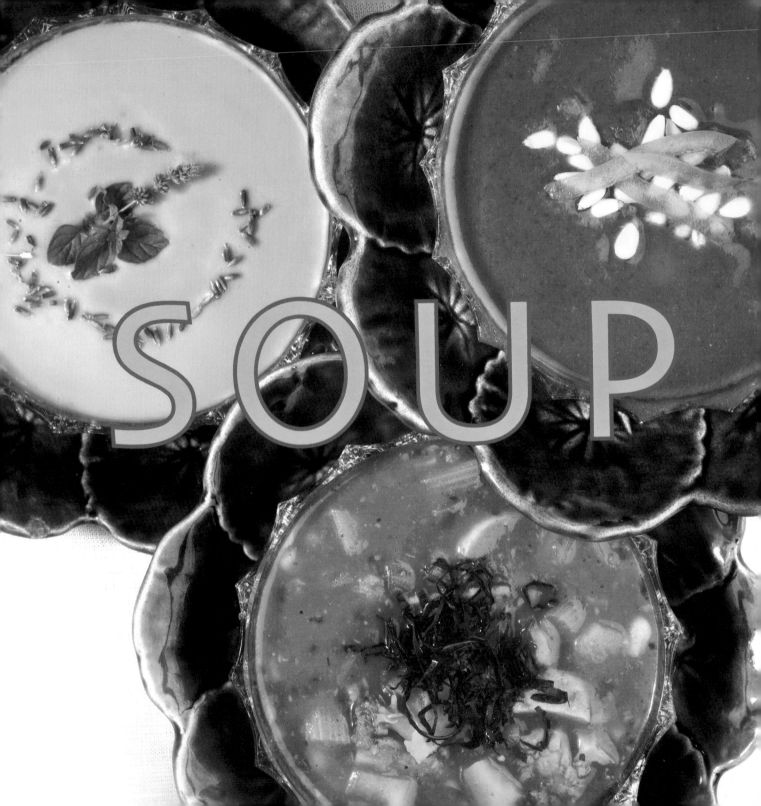

SOUP

VEGETABLE SOUP

1 or 2 cups of green celery tops, roughly chopped
1 medium potato, scrubbed and diced
1 medium carrot, diced
1 or 2 cups of any veggies you have on hand, such as green pepper, cauliflower, or broccoli, coarsely chopped
2 (15-ounce) cans stewed or diced tomatoes (preferably organic), or 2 or 3 large fresh tomatoes that are really ripe and good, seeded and chopped
1 medium onion, diced
½ cup dried lentils
Water to cover vegetables plus 1/3 more
1 cup frozen green peas—if you have fresh peas, so much the better
Pinch of sea salt or vegetable seasoning (such as Vegebase, Herbamare, or Spike)
1 tablespoon of fresh herb such as basil, thyme, or tarragon
1 tablespoon of extra virgin olive oil or non-dairy (vegan) butter

Put celery tops, potato, carrot, other veggies, lentils, and onion in a pot and add water until it covers all the veggies plus 1/3 more water.
Start on high heat. When water begins to boil, turn heat to medium, then low, and cover the pot.
Simmer gently until veggies begin to soften, about 20 minutes.
Put stewed tomatoes (or the fresh ones) into the blender and run on full speed just briefly (2 pulses). Add to the pot.
You don't want the soup to boil, but simmer gently until the vegetables are cooked through.
Add a cup of fresh or frozen green peas at this point.
Season to taste with salt or dried vegetable seasoning and add a fresh herb such as thyme, basil, or tarragon.
A tablespoon of buttery spread or extra virgin olive oil adds a fuller flavor.

I store extra soup in pint containers in the freezer for future quick lunches. A bowl of this soup, eaten before your green salad at night, with a slice of Avocado Treat makes for a hearty meal.

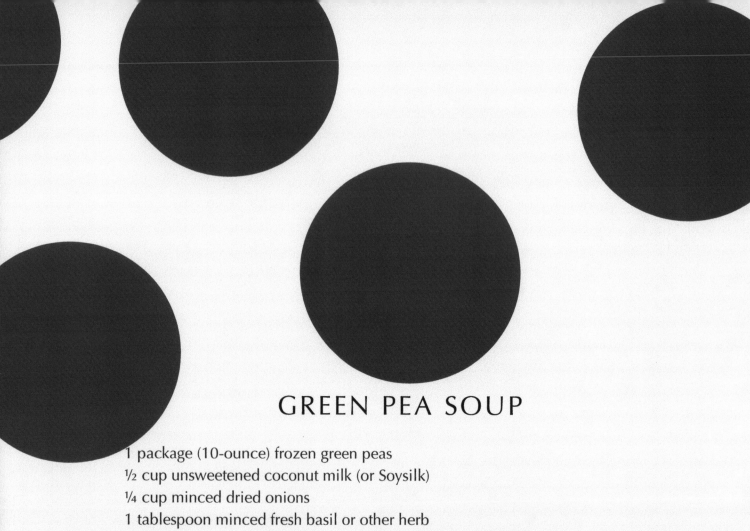

GREEN PEA SOUP

1 package (10-ounce) frozen green peas
½ cup unsweetened coconut milk (or Soysilk)
¼ cup minced dried onions
1 tablespoon minced fresh basil or other herb
Chopped sunflower seeds or almonds as a garnish

Steam peas until barely tender, about 4 or 5 minutes. Put peas in a blender with 2 or 3 cups boiling water; add the coconut or soymilk, minced onions, and sea salt or vegetable seasoning to taste. Blend on high speed until smooth. Add fresh basil or other herb of your choice, to taste. Serve piping hot with a garnish of chopped sunflower seeds or almonds, if you wish.

This recipe may be used substituting fresh or frozen broccoli or corn instead of peas. Delicious!

BEAN SOUP

3 cups dried beans, either black beans, white beans, or other varieties
1 can (15-ounce) tomato sauce
1 teaspoon ground cumin and/or chili seasoning, more or less to taste
3 tablespoons extra virgin olive oil

Soak the beans overnight, in twice as much water as beans.

Next day, drain and rinse the beans. This gets rid of much of the nitrogen gas, making for better digestion.

Put the beans in either a slow cooker, crock pot, or large stainless steel soup pot. Add 4 cups of water.

 I use a crock pot set on low—all you have to do is plug it in and leave it all day. It's a more gentle process and doesn't need as much attention. However, you can bring the beans to a boil on the stove in a soup pot, then lower the heat and simmer for about two hours, covered. Stir occasionally.

When the beans are soft (you may need to add more water midway through), add the tomato sauce, and cumin and/or chili seasoning to taste. Continue to simmer for 10–15 minutes as flavors combine.

Process half the soup mixture in a blender, adding the olive oil as you go along. Return mixture to the remainder of the soup to thicken it.

Any leftover soup can be frozen in pint-sized containers. It's easy to defrost for another meal or two later on.

CARROT GINGER SOUP

4 or 5 California carrots
1 Spanish onion
2 cups of water
Vegetable seasoning to taste
½ cup unsweetened coconut milk
2 tablespoons chopped fresh ginger root

Trim and slice the carrots.

Peel and slice the onion.

Place in a stainless steel pot with 2 cups of water. Start on high heat and lower the temperature when steam rises. Cover. In 7 or 8 minutes the carrots should be tender.

Pour the soup into the blender. Add seasoning to taste.

Add ½ cup of coconut milk and ginger, and blend on high, adding hot water as needed to get a smooth texture.

Serve piping hot.

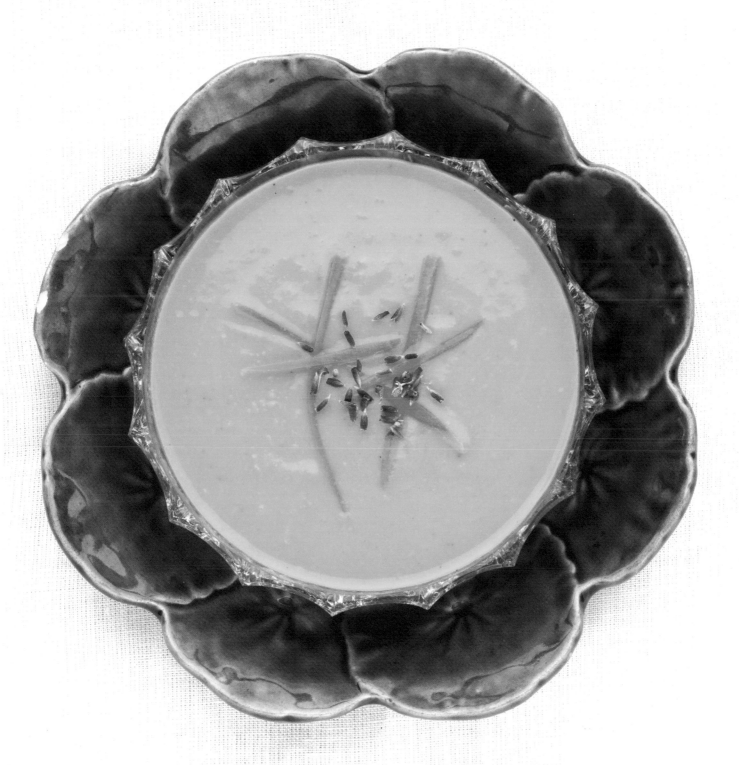

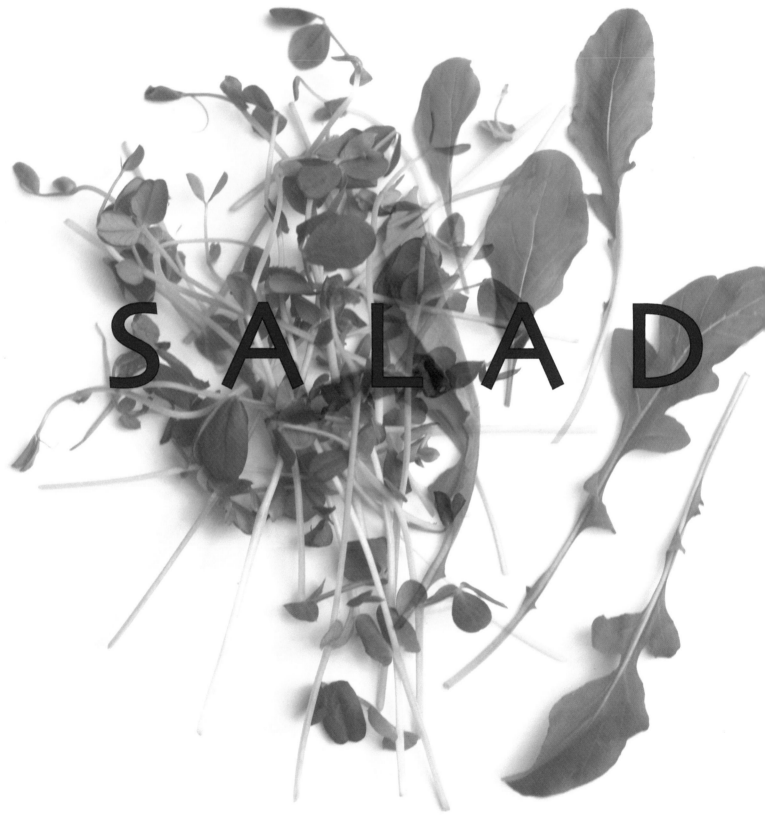

SALAD

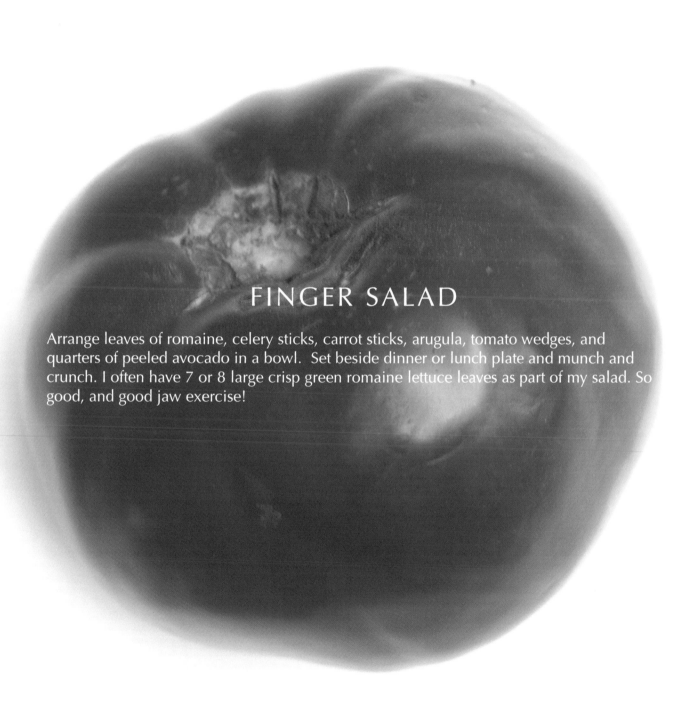

FINGER SALAD

Arrange leaves of romaine, celery sticks, carrot sticks, arugula, tomato wedges, and quarters of peeled avocado in a bowl. Set beside dinner or lunch plate and munch and crunch. I often have 7 or 8 large crisp green romaine lettuce leaves as part of my salad. So good, and good jaw exercise!

TOSSED GREEN SALAD

Medium-sized head of romaine lettuce
A few leaves of spinach or any other dark green leafy vegetable
About 1 tablespoon of extra virgin olive oil
About 1 tablespoon of fresh lemon juice
Vegetable seasoning or sea salt to taste

Tear the washed and dried leaves into bite-size pieces. Toss with a drizzle of olive oil, a few squirts of fresh lemon juice, and a sprinkling of vegetable seasoning.
Very often, instead of a mixed or tossed salad, I serve myself a dozen crispy dark green romaine lettuce leaves, and eat them au naturel. So good!

ARUGULA SALAD

2 or 3 generous handfuls of arugula leaves
About 1 teaspoon of extra virgin olive oil
About ½ teaspoon of fresh lemon juice
Vegetable seasoning or sea salt to taste

Toss washed and dried arugula leaves in a salad bowl with a light drizzle of olive oil, a dash of fresh lemon juice, and, if you wish, a pinch of salt or vegetable seasoning to taste.

Variations: add thin slices of cucumber and red pepper, and sprinkles of pine nuts or pumpkin seeds.

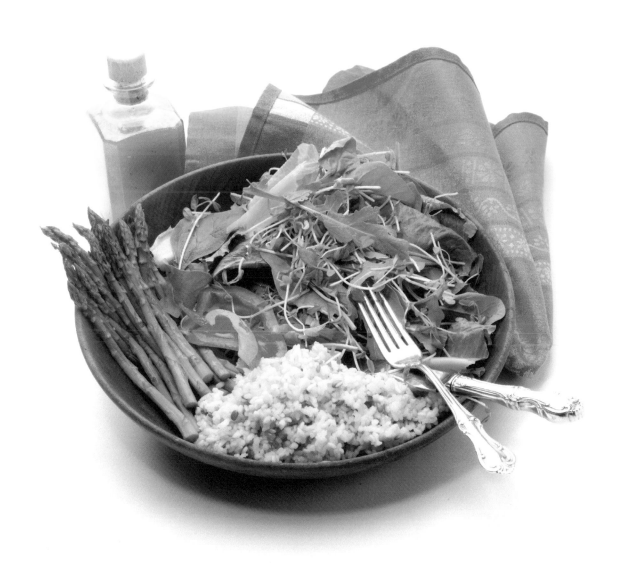

SPINACH SALAD

4 cups of spinach leaves
2 cups of Boston head lettuce, leaves torn apart
Handful of sprouts (any variety)
About 1 tablespoon of extra virgin olive oil
About 1 tablespoon of fresh lemon juice
Vegetable seasoning or sea salt to taste
2 tablespoons of pine nuts

Toss washed and dried greens together in salad bowl. Drizzle with olive oil, lemon juice, and a dusting of vegetable seasoning or a pinch of salt. Sprinkle in pine nuts.

RAINBOW SALAD

1 large California carrot
1 raw beet, peeled
½ head of romaine lettuce
8 leaves of Boston lettuce
3 or 4 plum tomatoes, sliced or chopped
1 ripe avocado, peeled and sliced
Joy's Basic Dressing (see recipe p. 70)

Grate the carrot and beet separately, either by hand or in your food processor. Thinly slice the washed and dried romaine leaves. Make a bed of the romaine in the serving bowl. Put a mound of grated carrots and a mound of beets (separately) on top. In between the mounds, place slices of the peeled avocado. Arrange Boston lettuce leaves around the edges, interspersed with the tomatoes. Drizzle with Joy's Basic Dressing.

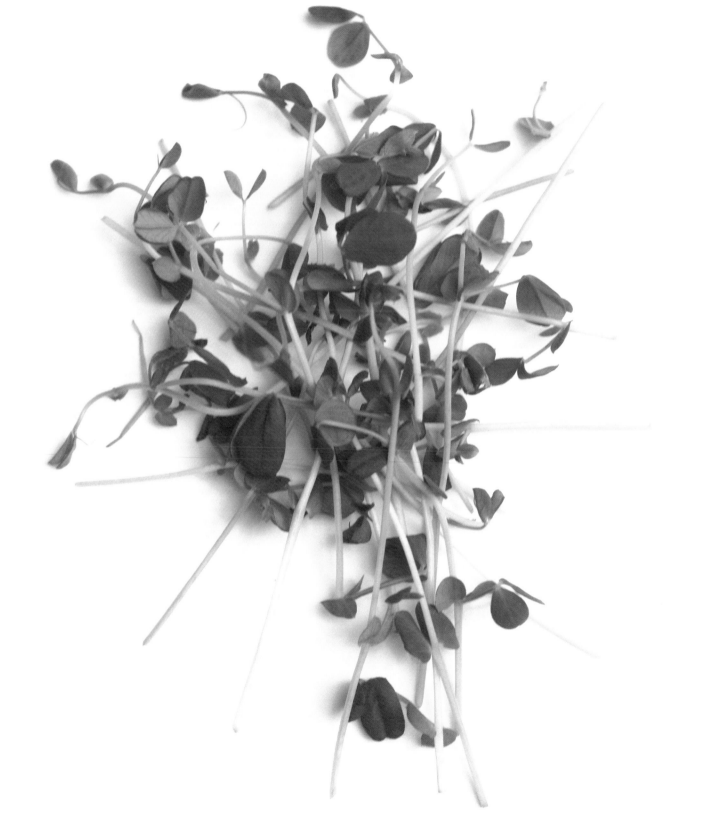

CARROT SALAD

3 or 4 medium-size California carrots
6 outside leaves of Boston lettuce
Joy's Pineapple Dressing (see recipe p. 71)

Grate the carrots, either by hand or in your food processor. Place 1 or 2 of the Boston lettuce leaves on each of the individual salad plates; then put a generous scoop of the grated carrots in the middle. Drizzle with the Pineapple Dressing. You might prefer to serve the dressing in a separate small pitcher and allow your family or guests to pour their own, to taste.

ANY LETTUCE SALAD

Check out the lettuces when you're doing your shopping. Look for the greenest and crispiest. Basic ones are romaine, arugula, spinach, and Boston. Keep lettuces washed, dried, and crispy in storage bags in your refrigerator crisper drawers, so all you have to do is pull out the bag and assemble the leaves into salad. With an assortment of sprouts, pre-made dressing (for example, Joy's Basic plus easily accessible extra virgin olive oil and your handy squirt bottle of fresh lemon juice and, for an occasional treat, a squirt bottle of balsamic vinegar) plus always available avocados, tomatoes, crunchy small cucumbers, Chinese snow pea pods, carrots, and green onions, you'll always have the makings for a large, satisfying salad as the best part of your dinner or lunch.

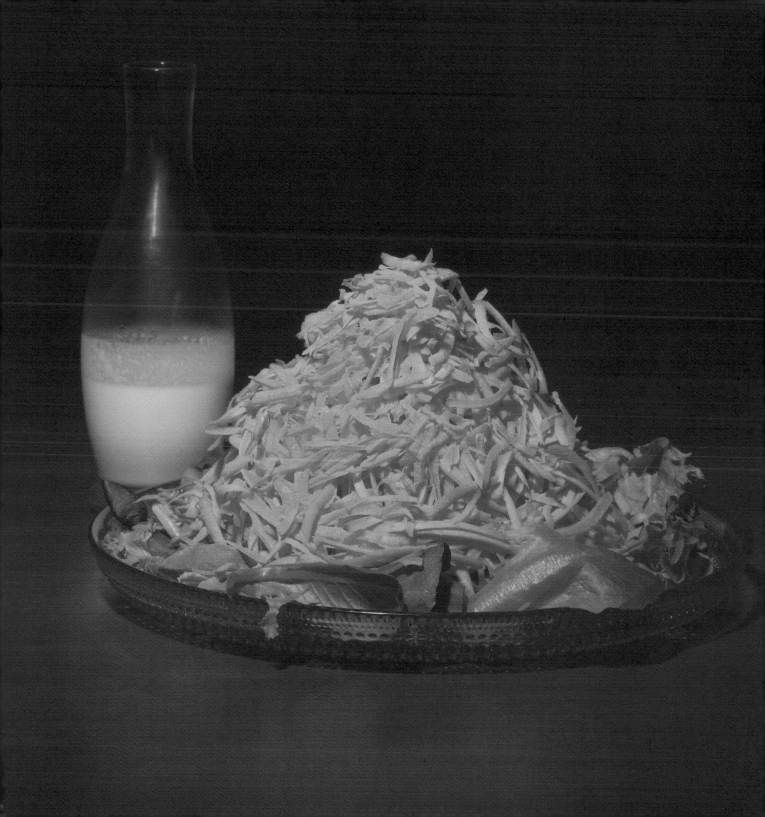

KALE SALAD WITH RAISINS

7 or 8 leaves of kale, washed and dried
2 tablespoons of chopped raisins
About 1 tablespoon of extra virgin olive oil
About 1 teaspoon of fresh lemon juice
About 1 tablespoon of finely diced apple (optional)
A few white grapes, thinly sliced (optional)

Kale is also a great staple. I prefer the Lacinato kale, which I get at my local health food store—but regular curly kale will be fine. Remove the ribs, lay the leaves flat, one on top of the other. Then roll tightly and slice very thinly with your chopping knife. Add the raisins and dress lightly with the olive oil and lemon juice. You may also add a tablespoon of finely diced apple or thinly sliced white grapes.

This is one of my very favorite salads, which I discovered at a great little restaurant, the Mercato, in nearby Red Hook. And the kale is loaded with all those blue-green phytonutrients such as calcium, amino acids, vitamins, and minerals, and the precious oxygen that alkalizes your cells. This is becoming my favorite salad. It tastes good, gives your jaws great exercise, and is so satisfying! I often double the recipe, and that's for one person—me! Yum.

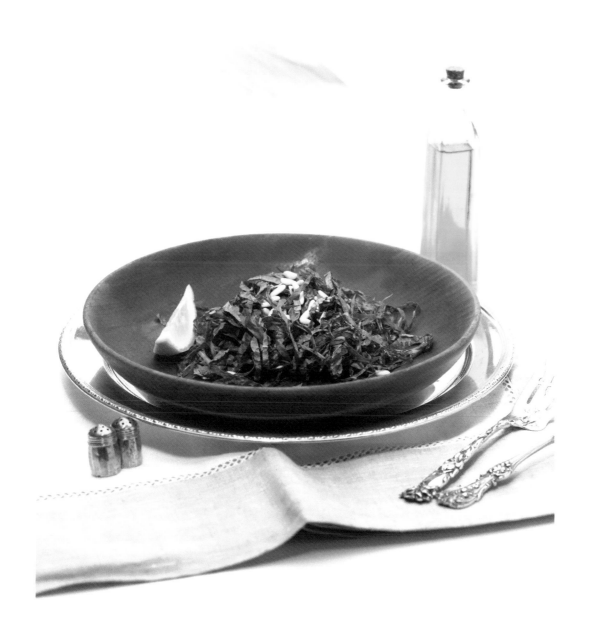

SALAD

Dressing

TOFUTTI SOUR CREAM DRESSING A LA JOY

This all-purpose soy-based dressing is also referred to as Joy's Tofutti Sour Cream.

    ½ cup Tofutti Sour Supreme (soy sour cream)
    2 or 3 tablespoons Soysilk or soy milk
    Vegetable seasoning or sea salt to taste
    1 teaspoon fresh lemon juice
    1 teaspoon dried minced onions
    A few leaves of your favorite herb, for example, basil or dill

Blend ingredients together on high speed In a blender or food processor. Adjust thickness by adding a little water if necessary to thin the dressing.

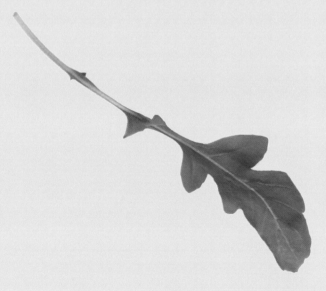

BASIC DRESSING

The basic way to dress a tossed green salad is to drizzle extra virgin olive oil and fresh lemon juice on the salad sparingly, to taste. Sprinkle lightly with vegetable seasoning and toss.

JOY'S CAESAR DRESSING

½ cup extra virgin olive oil
¼ cup fresh lemon juice
1 teaspoon Herbamare or vegetable seasoning of your choice
1 small clove garlic, peeled
1 teaspoon maple syrup or honey
¼ cup water

I am cautious with garlic. It contains a generous amount of mustard oil, which is irritating to the delicate membrane linings of your esophagus and digestive system. The residues, unwanted by your system, are sent back out via your breath, as they're not wanted inside of you. Thus, garlic breath!

Blend ingredients on high speed in a blender or food processor and store any leftovers in the refrigerator in a covered squirt bottle. You can easily double the recipe and store in a covered container in the fridge for handy future use.

AVOCADO DRESSING

1 ripe avocado, seeded and peeled
1 tablespoon peanut oil or other unsaturated vegetable oil
½ cup celery juice or tomato juice
1 teaspoon Herbamare or vegetable seasoning of your choice

Put all ingredients in a blender or food processor and combine until smooth. Add water if necessary for desired pourability.

JOY'S PINEAPPLE DRESSING

1/3 cup non-dairy (vegan) mayonnaise (for example, Vegenaise or Nayonaise)
Juice of ½ lemon
1 tablespoon of maple syrup
1 cup of unsweetened crushed and drained pineapple (or to taste)

Stir the lemon juice and maple syrup into the vegan mayonnaise until thoroughly mixed.
Add the crushed pineapple. This dressing is perfect with your
grated carrot salad or fresh sliced fruit.

Main Dish

YUMMY CHILI

2 cups pink beans (or black beans), soaked overnight in 4 cups of water, then drained, or 1 (15-ounce) can of beans, rinsed

1 small Spanish onion, chopped

2 cloves garlic, chopped

½ of a green bell pepper, chopped

1-½ cups of hydrolyzed soy protein (a special dispensation!)

1 tablespoon extra virgin olive oil

About 1 tablespoon chili powder (to taste)

Ground cumin, dried oregano, vegetable seasoning, or other herbs of your choice

1 (15-ounce) can of stewed tomatoes

1 cup tomato sauce

1 medium ripe fresh tomato, peeled and cubed (optional)

Cook dried beans in 4 cups of water, over low heat, until beans are tender (1-½ –2 hours).

In a large skillet, sauté onion, garlic, green pepper, and soy protein in olive oil until softened. Season to taste with chili powder and other herbs.

Lightly blend stewed tomatoes in food processor or blender, then add with tomato sauce to vegetable-soy mixture. Drain cooked beans and add to skillet. Simmer to blend flavors, about 15–20 minutes.

Transfer to serving bowl and drizzle with a little more olive oil if desired, for a richer flavor, and add cubed fresh tomato as a garnish.

AVOCADO TREAT

This is a treat I don't eat often but when I do, I really enjoy it. I use a seven-grain whole-wheat bread, which is made fresh daily at my nearby market. I buy it unsliced—it stays fresh longer that way, plus I can make the slices very thin if I choose. Half a loaf usually lasts me a month.

    2 slices whole-grain bread
    1 ripe avocado
    1 tablespoon onion, minced
    About 2 tablespoons celery or green bell pepper, chopped
    1 slice of tomato or roasted red pepper

Place two medium-thick slices of the bread on a plate.

Seed, peel, and mash the avocado. Mix in a tablespoon of minced onion, and if you wish, some chopped celery and/or green pepper.

Spread generously over the bread. Cut each slice into four pieces.

Top each one with a slice of fresh tomato or roasted red pepper.

This and a Green Smoothie will help you sail happily through until dinnertime!

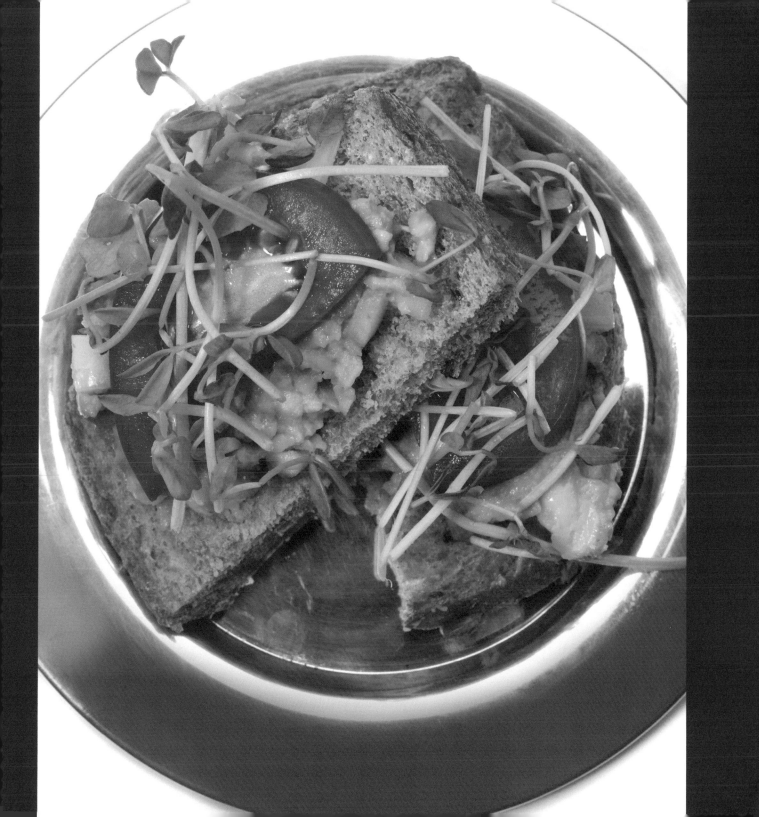

STUFFED PEPPERS

2 green or yellow or red bell peppers
2 cups steamed brown rice
1 tablespoon extra virgin olive oil
½ cup onion, minced
¼ cup celery, chopped
1 small garlic clove, peeled and minced
Vegetable seasoning or sea salt to taste
¼ cup of chopped fresh basil, or 1 teaspoon of dried basil
½ cup Tofutti Sour Supreme (soy sour cream)
Paprika and sprigs of arugula as a garnish

Preheat oven to 375 degrees.

Lightly steam the peppers in a covered saucepan until barely soft to the touch. Allow to cool, then halve each and remove the seeds, making 4 "cups" to stuff.

Sauté the garlic in the olive oil until soft but not browned, only a minute or so.

Add the minced onion and celery, seasoning as you go with a little sea salt or vegetable seasoning.

Add the steamed rice to the mixture, and ¼ cup of chopped fresh basil, or a teaspoon of dried basil.

Fold together with the Tofutti sour cream, and adjust the seasoning.

Spoon the filling evenly into the pepper halves; sprinkle lightly with paprika.

Arrange in a baking dish; cover with foil and heat in a 375-degree oven for about 25 minutes.

Garnish with sprigs of arugula just before serving.

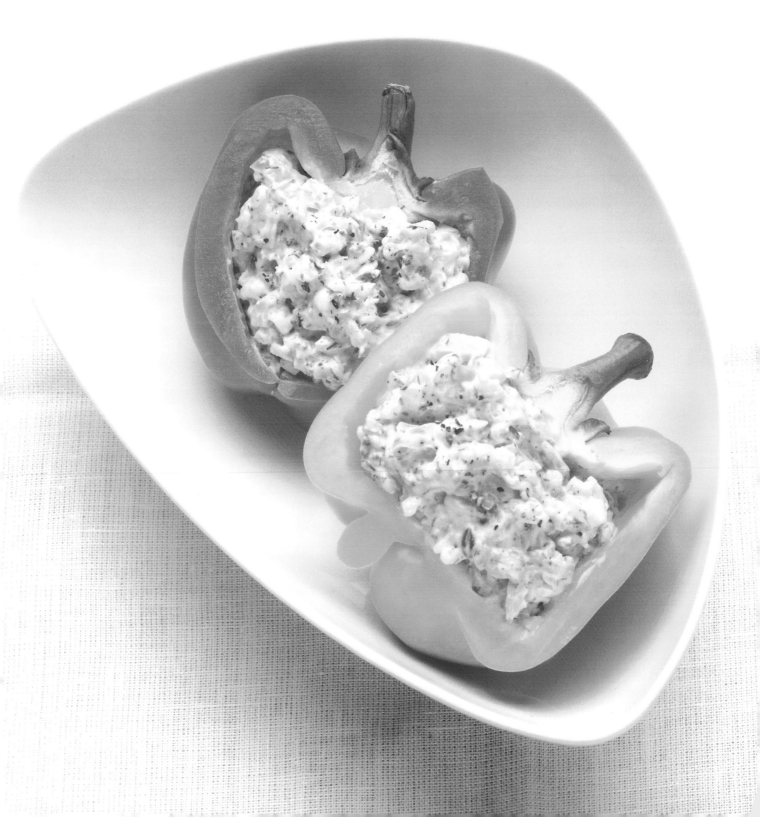

EGGPLANT SUPREME

1 medium-sized eggplant
¼ cup extra virgin olive oil
Vegetable seasoning to taste
1 small garlic clove, finely chopped, or 1/8 teaspoon garlic powder
Sprinkle of dried thyme (optional)
1-½ cups tomato or marinara sauce (preferably organic)
1 cup Tofutti Sour Supreme (soy sour cream)
1 teaspoon fresh lemon juice and a dash of soymilk (optional)
½ cup Tofutti mozzarella soy cheese, grated (or another brand)
Sprigs of arugula or fresh basil as a garnish

Preheat oven to 500 degrees with top rack in highest position.
Cut off both ends of eggplant. Cut into slices ½-inch thick. Place on a baking pan, which you've lightly coated with olive oil, then brush tops of slices generously with the olive oil. Sprinkle with vegetable seasoning and either finely chopped garlic or a very light sprinkle of garlic powder and dried thyme.
Place on the top rack in a 500-degree oven.
Brown on top, then turn the slices over and brown on the other side. Remove from pan.
Lower oven temperature to 400 degrees and lower rack to medium position.
Spread half the tomato sauce in the bottom of a baking dish, then place the eggplant slices on the sauce.
I stir in a teaspoon or so of fresh lemon juice and a dash of soymilk into the Tofutti sour cream to make it tastier, smoother, and lighter. Add a dollop of the Tofutti sour cream on top of each slice of eggplant.
Spoon the remainder of the tomato sauce generously on top of each slice, and sprinkle with the grated soy mozzarella.
Cover the dish loosely with foil and heat in a 400-degree oven for about 20 minutes, or until it begins to bubble around the edges.
Remove from the oven, remove foil, and add green sprigs of arugula, basil, or parsley around the edges and serve. This makes a nice company dish.

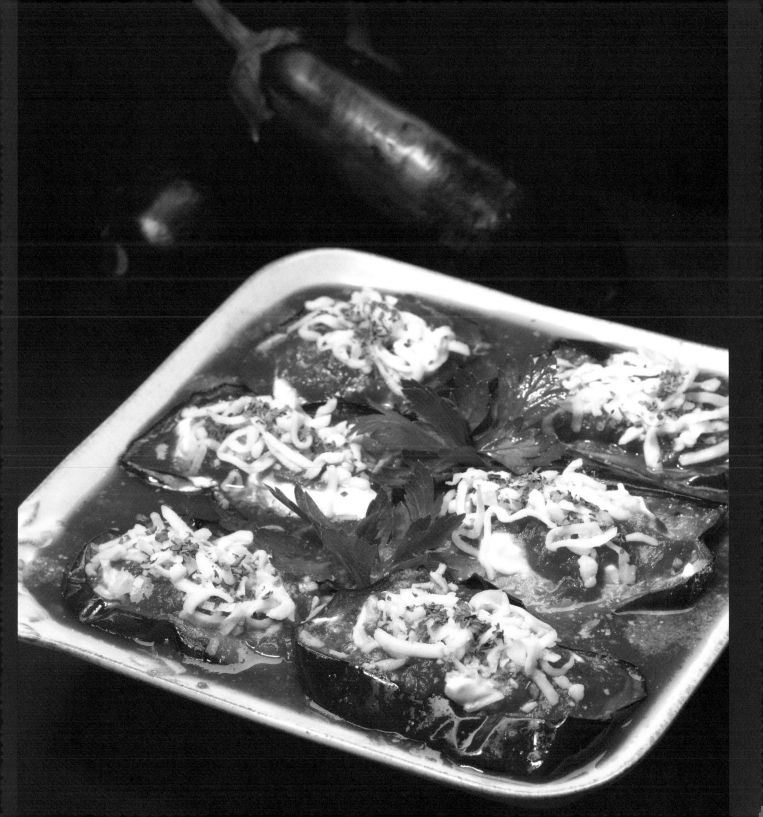

SQUASH A LA JOY

4 or 5 small to medium yellow summer squashes
1 Spanish onion
½ cup of water
7 or 8 Chinese snow pea pods
Vegetable seasoning or sea salt to taste
About 1 teaspoon dried dill
1 tablespoon buttery spread (vegan)

Remove ends from squashes and cut into thick slices.

Peel and slice onion.

Place both in a stainless steel saucepan with a tight-fitting cover. Add ½ cup of water.

 Cook on high until the steam begins to rise, then cover and steam on medium-low heat for about 10 minutes, or until just tender.

At the last minute put the snow peas in the pan and replace the lid. This barely steams the pods and adds green and flavor to the dish.

Remove the snow peas to another dish and put half the squash in the blender.

Add the buttery spread, a pinch or so of vegetable seasoning, and a teaspoon or so of dried dill to taste. Blend until smooth.

Coarsely mash the squash that remains in the pan.

Combine the blender squash with the mashed squash, add the snow peas, and serve. You can also put the mashed squash and snow peas in the bowl and ladle the blender squash on top as a sauce.

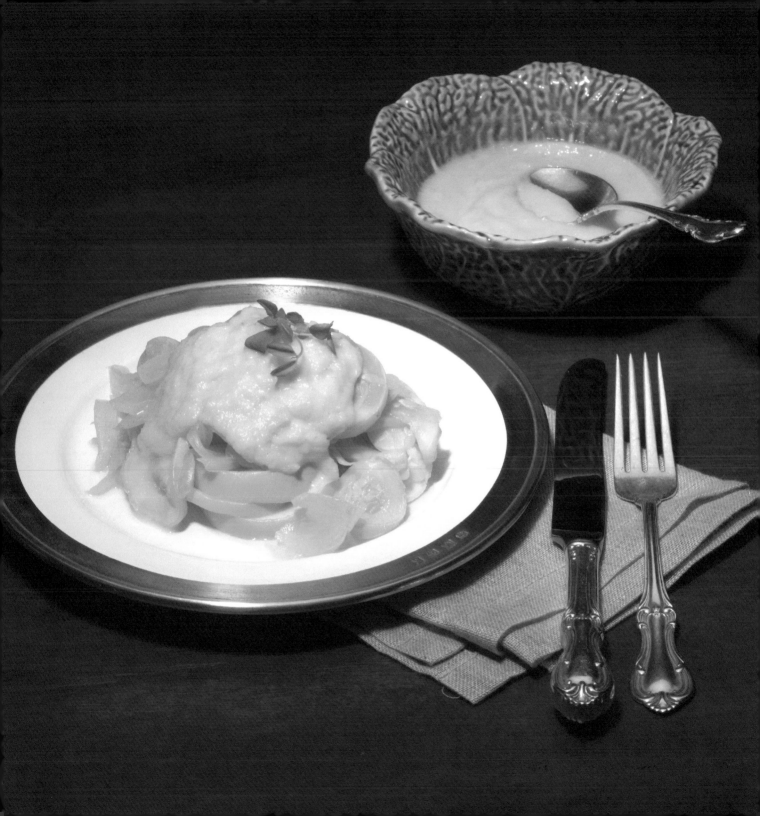

CHINESE STIRFRY

2 tablespoons extra virgin olive oil
1 medium clove garlic, minced
1 cup each of carrots, celery, zucchini, and onion, cut into strips about 2 inches long
1 cup Chinese snow pea pods, sliced lengthwise
1 block of firm tofu, cut into strips
2 or 3 cups mung bean sprouts
3 cups steamed brown rice
Drizzle of Bragg's Liquid Aminos (or soy sauce)

I like to use my stainless steel electric pan for this stirfry dish, although a regular nonstick skillet or other sauté pan will do just fine.
Drizzle the olive oil into the pan. Add the garlic, stirring until it begins to brown around the edges. Then add other ingredients, ending with the sprouts. When the steam starts to rise, cover and turn heat to low. The dish should be just perfect in 10 minutes.
Before serving over brown rice, drizzle lightly with the Bragg's or soy sauce.

RICE CONFETTI

2-½ cups water
1 cup short grain or sticky brown rice
1 cup arborio rice
¼ cup wheat berries
sea salt or vegetable seasoning (optional)
slices of roasted red peppers
slices of peeled avocado
fresh basil leaves as garnish

I use my small rice steamer for this recipe, although the same directions can be followed for cooking in a covered saucepan.
Put the water and the rices and wheat berries in the steamer pot. Bring to a boil with heat on high. After 5 or 6 minutes turn to low, and cover with lid. Leave it sit for 45 minutes, as it will continue to absorb water and steam. Before serving, turn under and over gently with a fork to mix the rices. Serve as individual portions, topped with roasted red peppers and chunky slices of avocado and a garnish of fresh basil leaves. This mixed rice also is delicious just as it is, without the garnishes. It's also super good topped with with any kind of beans, tomato sauce, or a good salsa. This and a large green salad make a satisfying meal.

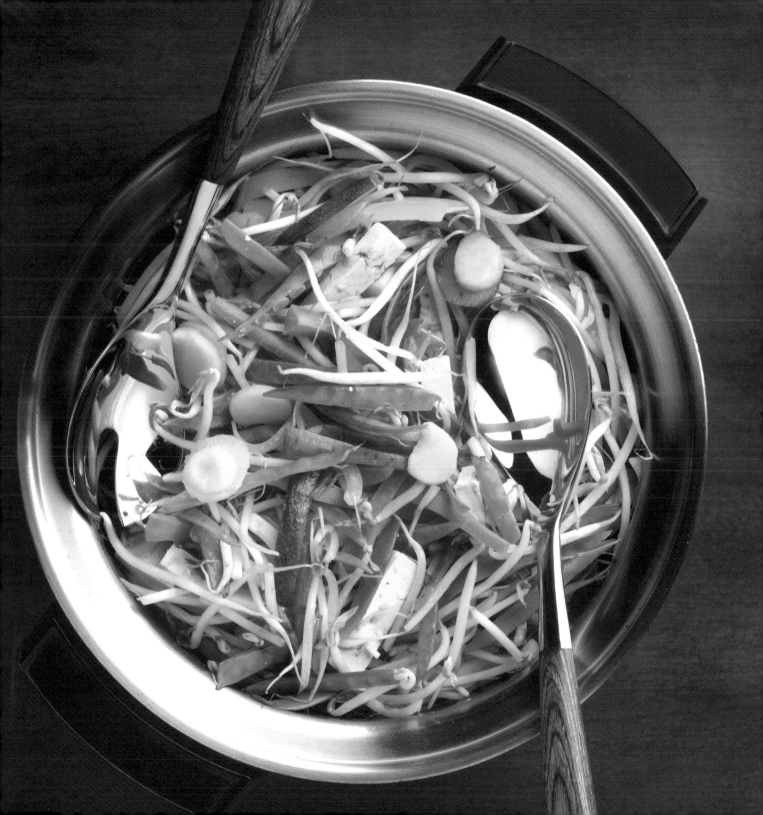

LUSCIOUS LINGUINI

1 package (12–16 ounce) whole-wheat linguini

1 (15-ounce) can crushed tomatoes, preferably organic, or 3 fresh ripe tomatoes, peeled, cored, and chopped or crushed

 2 tablespoons extra virgin olive oil

1 clove elephant garlic, peeled and chopped (not as strong as regular)

1 small white onion, chopped

1 green bell pepper, seeded and chopped (or Italian frying pepper)

Handful of fresh basil leaves, chopped

1 tablespoon fresh oregano, chopped, or ½ teaspoon dried oregano

Sea salt, to taste

1 cup tomato juice, if needed to thin sauce (optional)

Tofutti mozzarella soy cheese, grated, or grated Parmesan-flavor soy cheese (optional)

In a large skillet, sauté garlic, onion, and green pepper in the olive oil. Add basil and oregano. Add tomatoes and incorporate into the sautéed ingredients. Adjust seasoning to taste.

Meanwhile, cook the linguini according to instructions on the package. Lift the pasta from the cooking water to the sauce in the skillet. Swirl together gently. You may want to add a cup of tomato juice if needed for more "slurpidity."

Serve right from the pan, or transfer to a large serving bowl in the center of the table, or onto individual plates. Grated tofu mozzarella or soy cheese topping may be passed around for final touch.

Arugula Salad would be a perfect accompaniment.

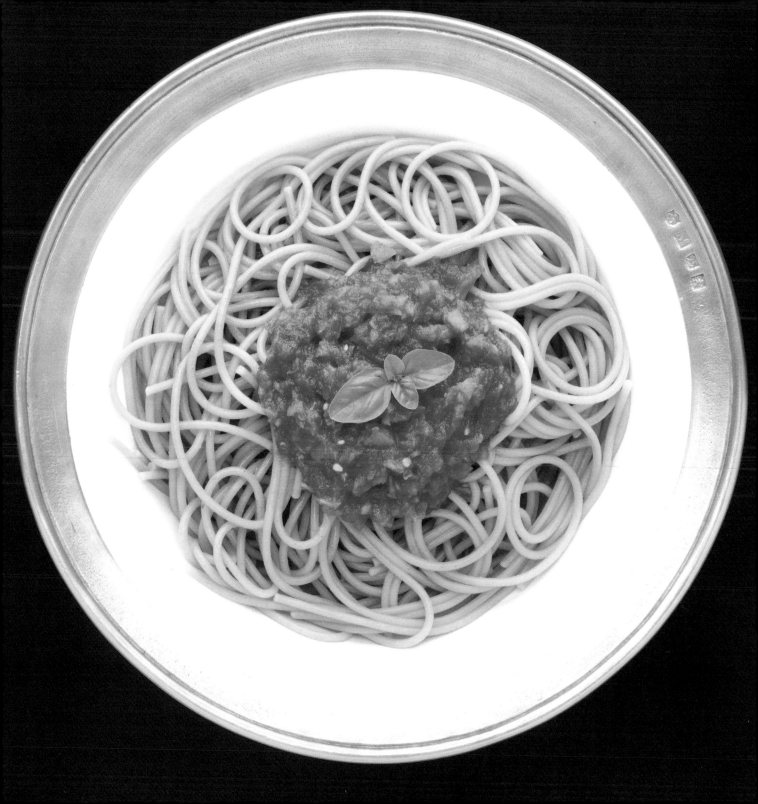

BROCCOLI DIVINE

1 head of broccoli, separated into florets
1/3 cup of water
2 tablespoons of extra virgin olive oil
1 small clove garlic or ½ clove of elephant garlic, peeled and minced
4 or 5 medium white mushrooms, sliced
2 teaspoons of fresh lemon juice
Sea salt to taste
¾ cup Tofutti mozzarella soy cheese, shredded

Preheat oven to 350 degrees.

Pour about 1/3 cup of water into a saucepan with a tight-fitting cover. Lightly steam the broccoli by starting on high heat; when steam rises, cover the pan and turn heat to low.

Steam for 4 or 5 minutes. Broccoli should be tender but very firm and bright green.

In a sauté pan lightly brown the garlic (do not burn) and mushrooms in the olive oil until just golden.

Arrange the broccoli and mushrooms in an ovenproof serving dish; add the lemon juice and seasoning. Spread the cheese over the top; melt in oven at 350 degrees for 5 minutes. Serve immediately.

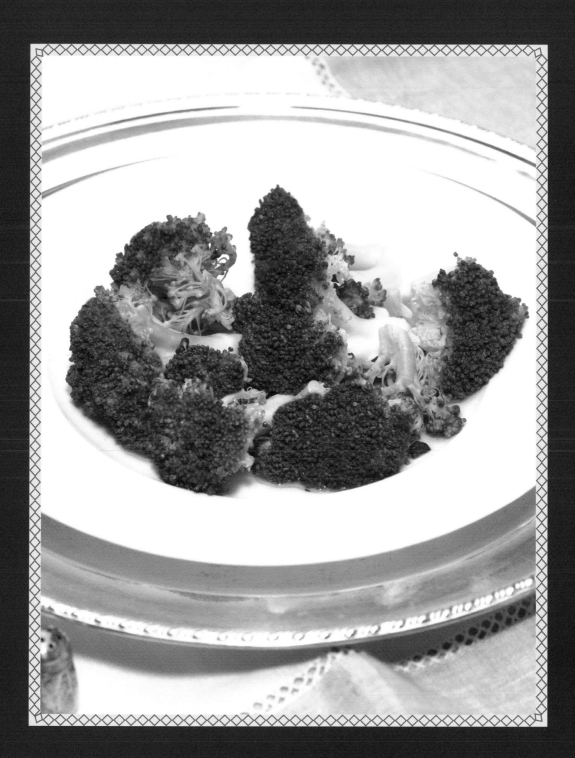

QUESADILLA TREAT

4 whole-grain tortillas

2 teaspoons extra virgin olive oil

1 cup cooked pink beans (rinsed if canned)

½ Vidalia onion

1 tablespoon chili seasoning or to taste

1 cup tomato sauce, plus another ¼ cup as a garnish

1 tablespoon fresh lemon juice

Sea salt to taste

1 avocado, seeded, peeled, and diced

Handful of green pea sprouts as a garnish

Chopped black olives and tomato as a garnish

½ cup Joy's Tofutti Sour Cream (see recipe p. 69)

Place all ingredients (except the tortillas, olive oil, avocado, and garnishes) in a food processor or blender and process until smooth. Adjust consistency by adding a little more tomato sauce if needed.

Heat the olive oil in a sauté pan; cook each tortilla flat in the pan until soft with a hint of golden on both sides.

Place the warm tortillas flat on your work surface. Spoon 1 tablespoon of tomato sauce in a line down the middle of each tortilla. Add ¼ of the blended bean mixture, and then bring sides together to form a roll. Spoon tomato sauce on top, add the diced avocado, and top with a teaspoon of Joy's Tofutti Sour Cream and green pea shoots, olives, or tomato as a garnish. (Alternatively, you can choose to add the avocado and garnishes inside the tortilla before rolling.) Serve on a pretty plate with a fork and a small sharp knife.

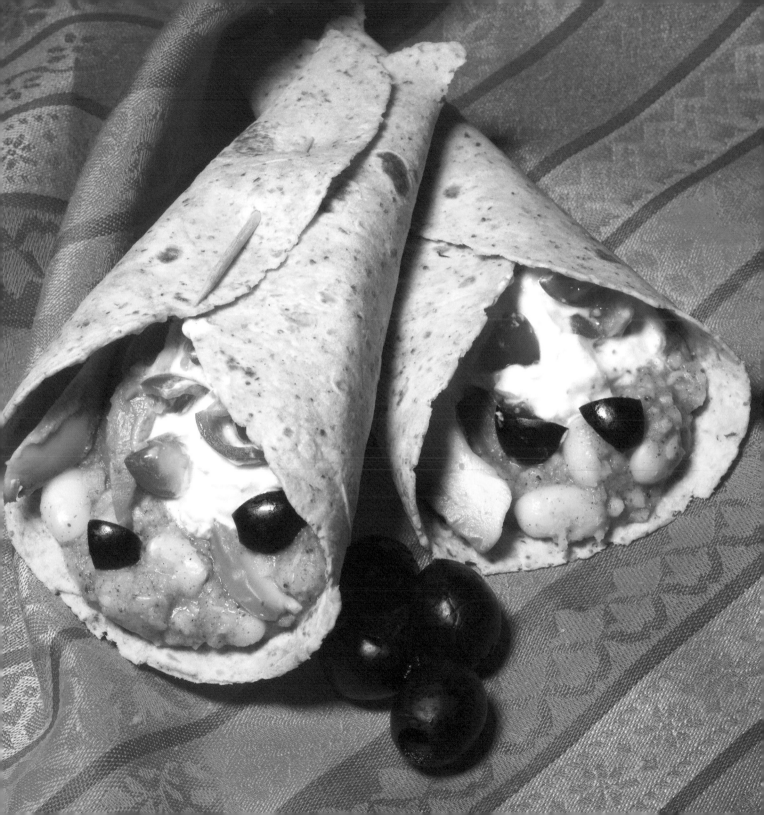

POLENTA

5 cups water

1 cup organic corn grits or coarse cornmeal (polenta)

½ teaspoon sea salt

½ teaspoon finely chopped fresh thyme

¼ cup extra virgin olive oil

1 green bell pepper, seeded and thinly sliced

1 small white onion, peeled and thinly sliced

1 cake organic baked tofu (about 2 ounces), cut into thin strips

1 small clove garlic, peeled and thinly sliced

1 or 2 pinches red pepper flakes (optional, to taste)

½ cup black olives, drained

Bring the water to a boil in a deep skillet. Add the seasoning and thyme, and then pour in the polenta in a thin stream, stirring all the while on a lower heat. When the polenta becomes thick and smooth, pour into an 8-inch by12-inch baking dish. Smooth the top with a spoon and let cool.

Meanwhile, process the olives in a food processor or chopper until pulverized.

Heat the olive oil in a sauté pan. Lightly brown the green pepper, onion and tofu, adding red pepper flakes if desired. Add garlic and toss lightly until golden. Remove from heat.

Turn the polenta upside down on your work surface; cut it into rectangles, then each rectangle in half. Arrange in a baking dish.

Spread the olives evenly on top of each piece; then spoon on the veggies. Serve hot. You may also heat the polenta first, then spoon the hot veggies over the top on individual plates.

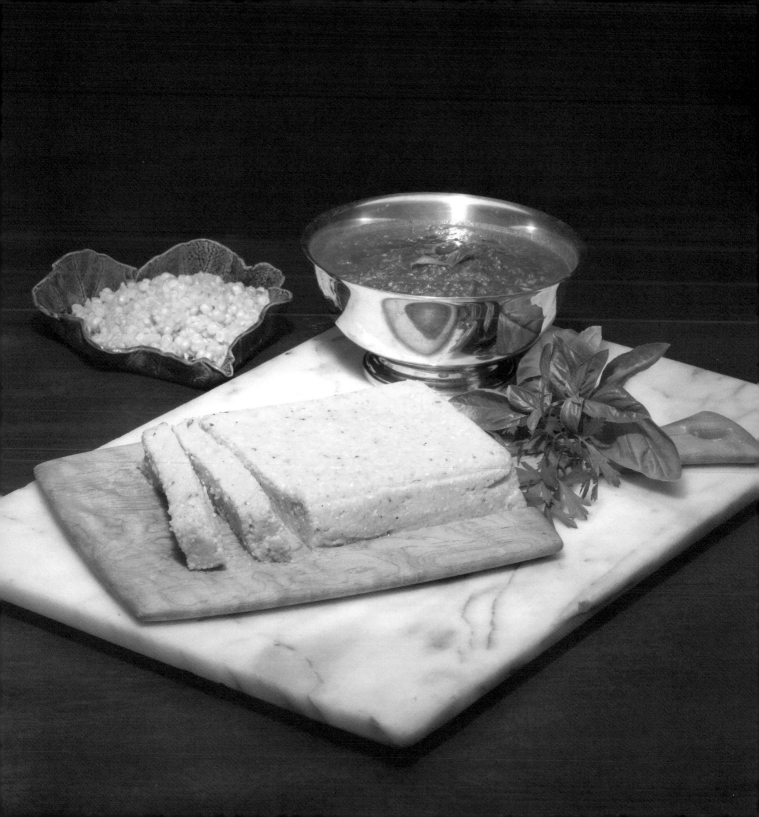

POTATOES ANNA A LA JOY

3 medium Idaho (baking) potatoes
½ cup coconut cream
Vegetable seasoning or sea salt to taste
Arugula or parsley leaves as a garnish.

Preheat oven to 450 degrees.

Thinly peel the potatoes, and then slice each one about ¼ inch thick.

Select a round baking dish that can also be used directly on the stovetop. An enameled baking pan or cast-iron skillet is a good choice.

Pour half of the coconut cream in the bottom of the pan. Start cooking on high heat; as the cream melts, swish it evenly around the bottom of dish.

Place the potato slices evenly, flat, on the bottom. Traditionally the slices are placed in an overlapping spiral, beginning at the center of the pan. Sprinkle the seasoning lightly over all, then put a tablespoon of the cream on each slice. Repeat layering until all potatoes are in place.

When the bottom layer is browned at the edges (check with a spatula), place the pan in the oven at 450 degrees and bake for about 45 minutes, or until slightly brown on top.

Remove from the oven. Place a plate on top of the pan and invert it, so the potatoes form a "cake" on the plate. You may need to slide a spatula underneath to insure safe delivery.

Garnish with fresh herbs such as arugula or parsley.

You may also serve extra coconut cream on the side for anyone who may wish it.

I use the canned organic coconut milk, which is available at health food stores. It basically is more like a cream, especially the concentrated kinds that have higher fat (oil) content.

I only make this for special occasions, as it's more work than I want to perform for myself.

GREEN BEAN SPECIAL

2 medium white onions, peeled and sliced
2/3 cup dried porcini mushrooms, soaked in water for at least an hour. Remove from water; remove stems and slice each mushroom lengthwise once.
About 1-½ pounds of fresh green beans, washed and trimmed
½ cup water
 Vegetable seasoning to taste.
1 tablespoon extra virgin olive oil
Joy's Basic Dressing

Select beautiful, long slender green beans—the amount you'll need for the number of guests you'll be having. The quantity suggested above will serve four people.

Soak the dried porcini mushrooms in water to cover for at least an hour. Remove from water, cut off stems, and slice each mushroom lengthwise once.

Heat olive oil in a sauté pan, and add the sliced onions. Cook until golden and soft, then add the porcini mushrooms and cook gently for about 5–6 minutes. Remove from heat.

Place the green beans in a steamer or sauté pan, with ¼ cup water for steaming. Sprinkle with vegetable seasoning to taste. Start heat on high. When steam begins to rise, turn to low and cover with a tight-fitting lid. Only 5 minutes should do it!

Carefully place the beans on a serving plate. Arrange onions and mushrooms around the outside of the beans, and drizzle with Joy's Basic Dressing (see recipe p. 70).

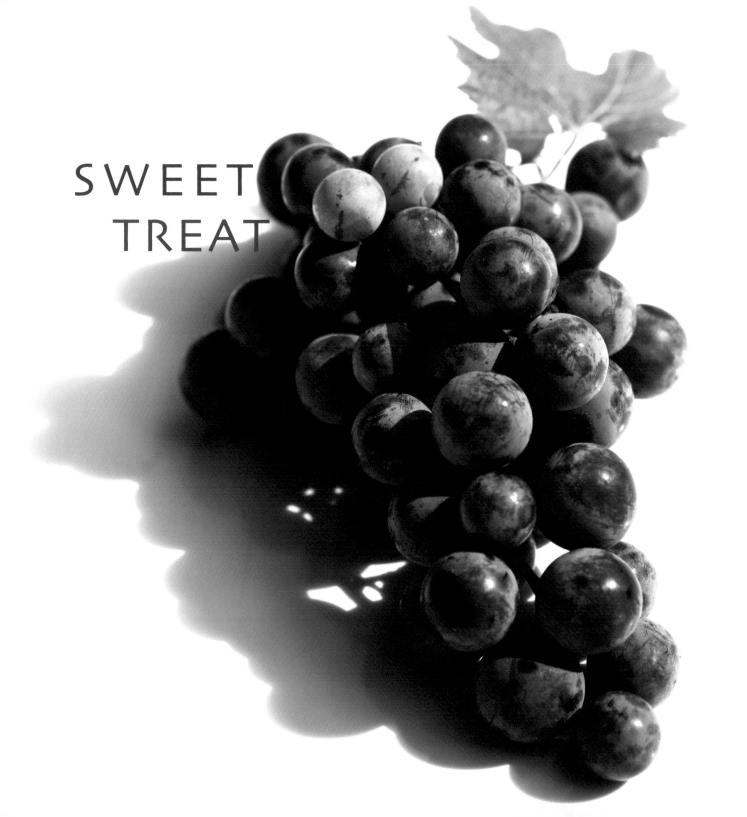

SWEET
TREAT

CASHEW BUTTER BALLS

I make my own cashew butter, using my Champion juicer. It's sooo versatile! I insert a blank slide attachment instead of the porous screen you'd use for juicing.

I buy my cashews at my local health food store—raw—and keep them in the freezer. But before using them for this purpose, I leave them out overnight, as they go through the juicer more easily when thawed. Make the butter at least a day before you make the Cashew Butter Balls. The butter won't work when warm, because it has to thicken.

2 cups raw cashews
Drizzles of safflower or canola oil, if needed for smoother flow
Pinch of sea salt
2 teaspoons of maple syrup
Halves of green grapes as a garnish

Put the cashews through the feeder in small batches, about ¼ cup each, until they're finished. Scoop into a bowl, add the pinch of salt and the maple syrup, and stir to incorporate thoroughly.

Store the butter in a pint container in the fridge so it will become more solid, like butter, instead of being runny. You need to do all this at least a day before you make the balls.

The next day, use a melon baller to scoop out the cashew balls. Wow!

Arrange them on a pretty plate. Top some of them with halves of green grapes and leave some plain. Stick a toothpick in the top center of each one. Add a fresh flower for oomph. I use my own hibiscus—in season, of course—as an accent on the edge of the plate.

And there you have it!

BANANA COCONUT CREAM PIE

2 large or 3 medium ripe bananas, sliced
10 plump medjool or khadrawi dates
1-½ cup Joy's Vanilla Crème (see recipe p.103)
2 large kiwis, peeled and sliced
2 or 3 large strawberries, hulled and sliced
1 ripe mango, peeled and sliced (ripe peach may be substituted)
Unsweetened shredded coconut
Handful of fresh blueberries

The bananas should be completely ripe, speckled with brown. Halve the dates, remove seeds, and press them cut side down to cover the bottom of a pie plate. Arrange banana slices generously over the dates.

Cover with the Vanilla Crème, then sprinkle shredded coconut generously over the crème. Tuck sliced kiwi and strawberries around the edge. Or use sliced mango instead and arrange the strawberries across the top. Half a sliced blueberry placed in the center of the strawberry slice looks pretty.

This has always been a big hit at my food demonstrations.

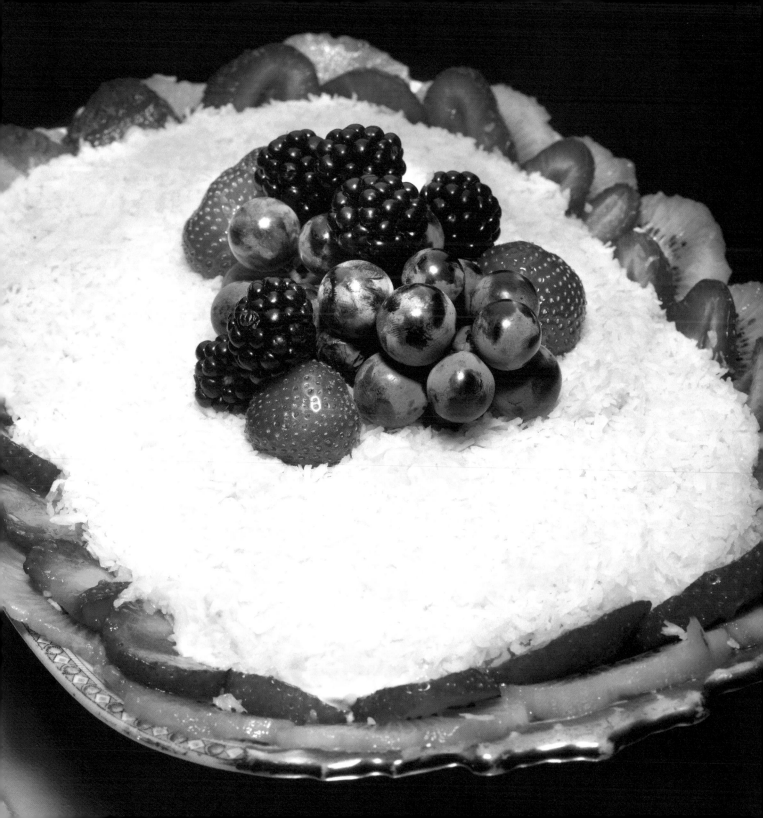

FIVE-FRUIT SUNDAE

This dessert could just as well be a three-fruit sundae. These five fruits work nicely together, although you may choose others.

    5 or 6 strawberries, hulled and sliced
    ¼ cup of blueberries
    ¼ cup of raspberries small ripe banana, sliced
    1 kiwi, peeled and sliced
    2/3 cup Joy's Vanilla Crème (see recipe p. 103)
    Sprig of mint leaves as a garnish

In a tall crystal or glass goblet, starting with the crème on the bottom, layer the fruit in separate layers between spoonfuls of the crème, finishing with a strawberry and a sprig of mint on top. Indulge your own artistry!

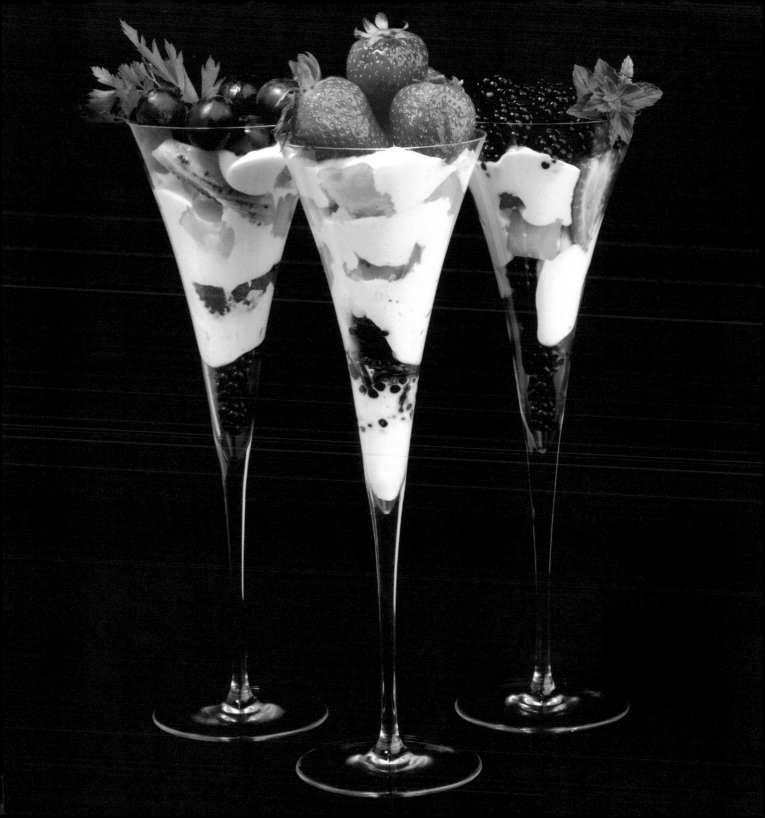

MANGO TREAT

1 ripe mango
Handful of Bing cherries
Small bunches of white seedless grapes

Cut a ripe mango in half, slicing around the large flat seed in the middle to remove it.

With a sharp paring knife, score the flesh of the mango into cubes, being careful not to cut through the skin. Arrange each half cut side up on an oval plate, along with some Bing cherries and small bunches of white seedless grapes.

This treat is not only delicious but beautiful as well. One mango makes two portions for dessert. You can also serve this as a yummy lunch, one mango per person.

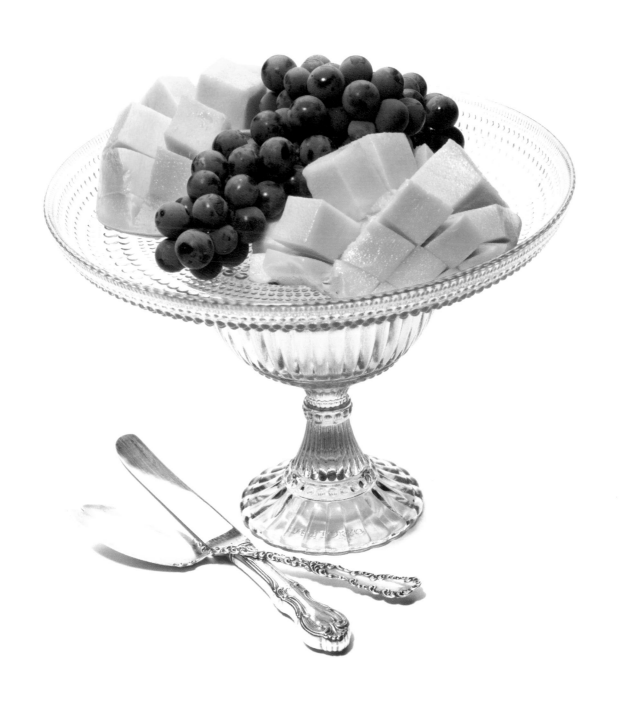

VERY SPECIAL ORANGE CAKE

8 ounces non-dairy (vegan) unsalted butter at room temperature
1- ¼ cup of granulated brown sugar
5-ounce chunk of firm organic tofu
3 tablespoons of orange zest
1/3 cup of fresh-squeezed orange juice
1-½ cups of whole-wheat pastry flour
¼ teaspoon baking powder
¼ teaspoon baking soda
½ teaspoon kosher salt
1/3 cup soy buttermilk
½ teaspoon vanilla extract

Preheat oven to 350 degrees.
Put all the ingredients in a food processor or a blender and process until smooth. Pour into a 9-inch round cake pan that has been lightly greased with vegan butter and lightly floured.
Bake for 40–45 minutes at 350 degrees or until a cake tester comes out clean. Let cool for 10–15 minutes. Remove from pan and place on a baking rack.
Spoon glaze (see below) over the cake and allow to cool. When the glaze is dry, wrap well and store in freezer until ready for that very special occasion (or serve immediately if that occasion is today!). A touch of Joy's Vanilla Crème (see recipe p. 103) or Chocolate Pudding (see recipe p. 107) might be spooned atop each slice as served.

FOR BUTTERMILK:

1/3 cup of Soysilk or soy milk
4 or 5 squirts of fresh lemon juice

Stir well. The lemon juice will act upon the soy milk. Voilà! Buttermilk.

FOR GLAZE:

½ cup maple syrup
1 tablespoon fresh-squeezed orange juice

Combine until smooth and spoon over the cake.
I use this recipe for special occasions, usually a birthday dinner or party.

JOY'S VANILLA CRÈME

½ cup Tofutti Sour Supreme (soy sour cream)
½ cup Joy's Cashew Butter (see recipe p. 95)
1 tablespoon fresh lemon juice
¼ cup of maple syrup (or to taste)
2 tablespoons of coconut cream
1 teaspoon of vanilla extract

Combine all ingredients in a blender until smooth. I store this lovely topping in a squirt bottle in the refrigerator, where it's always handy to lend a special touch to fresh fruit or other desserts.

DRIED FRUIT CONFECTION

15 plump medjool or khadrawi dates

2/3 cups raisins

12 soft dried prunes

About ¼ cup of maple syrup

 2 heaping tablespoons of cashew or peanut butter (unprocessed and unsalted, preferably homemade)

1-½ cups unsweetened shredded coconut

I use my Champion juicer to pulverize the dried fruits. You may use a meat grinder or your
food processor. I actually mix my dried fruits on my wooden cutting board, but you can
transfer the dried fruit to a bowl. Then incorporate the maple syrup and the cashew or
peanut butter.

Roll into marble-sized round balls, and then roll those in coconut. Store them in the
freezer for future happy treats for kids and grownups alike.

BANANA ICE CREAM AND PINEAPPLE SORBET

Only the Champion juicer has the ability to make ice cream, sherbet, or sorbet, to my knowledge.

3 ripe bananas, with a few brown speckles
Maple syrup for drizzling
Sprig of mint as a garnish

Place peeled bananas in airtight zip-lock storage bags in the freezer—at least overnight.

Remove from the freezer and feed through the Champion juicer, using the blank slide attachment instead of the screen one you'd use for juicing.

Voilà, there's your ice cream. Serve in pretty dessert bowls or goblets. Drizzle with maple syrup and garnish with a sprig of mint.

YOU CAN ALSO MAKE DELICIOUS PINEAPPLE SORBET, IN THE SAME MANNER.

1 ripe pineapple
Crystallized raw sugar
Kiwi, peeled and sliced, as a garnish

Simply peel and core a ripe pineapple and cut into thick strips. Cut the strips into chunks and freeze in a ziplock storage bag, at least overnight.

Feed through the Champion juicer, using the blank slide attachment.

Serve in stemmed wine glasses (for very special!) or pretty small bowls. Sprinkle with a dusting of crystallized raw sugar and garnish with a slice of peeled kiwi.

DATE DELIGHT

12 plump medjool or khadrawi dates
24 large walnut halves
fresh mint leaves as a garnish

These are large, sweet, and luscious types of dates. I like the khadrawi dates better, but they are more difficult to find.

Split each date in half, removing seeds as you do so. Stuff a large walnut half in the center of each date half. Arrange on a pretty plate, garnished with mint leaves. You can make fewer halves, depending on your guest list.

AMBROSIA

6 Honeybell oranges
Joy's Vanilla Crème (see recipe p. 103)
Unsweetened shredded coconut

Peel the oranges and cut into wedges, going around the core, thus sidetracking the center seed area. Arrange the orange wedges in pretty glass or crystal small dishes, and garnish with Joy's Vanilla Crème and the shredded coconut.

CHOCOLATE PUDDING

2 ripe avocados (firm but not hard), seeded, peeled, and diced
¼ cup of maple syrup
¼ cup plus 2 tablespoons coconut butter (or coconut cream)
¼ cup of cacao powder
1/3 cup water
1 teaspoon of vanilla extract
Mint leaves as a garnish

Put all ingredients into a food processor or a blender. Process until nice and creamy.

Transfer to fancy Champagne glasses and garnish with a mint leaf.

Special thanks to my friend Hillary Huntington for this divine recipe, which—even though I use it infrequently, usually for company—I thoroughly enjoy.

INDEX TO RECIPES